Swimming Pools

Swimming Pools

A HomeOwner's Bible

PETER JONES

DOUBLEDAY & COMPANY, INC., GARDEN CITY, NEW YORK 1982

ACKNOWLEDGMENTS

The author gratefully acknowledges the following persons, companies, and associations for their contributions toward the creation of this book:

The National Swimming Pool Institute, 200 K Street, N.W., Washington, D.C. 20006, for the many excellent pictures and invaluable information provided to the author.

The Hayward Manufacturing Company, Inc., 900 Fairmont Avenue, Elizabeth, N.J. 07207, for the photographs and drawings of all pool accessories shown in the book.

Mr. Charles R. Gaglio, President of St. G Pools, Inc., 49 North Union Street, Lambertville, N.J. 08530, for both the technical information and advice during the construction of a Gunite pool, which his company was building.

Mr. and Mrs. James Mazza, for their patience and cooperation while the author photographed the construction of their in-ground pool.

Library of Congress Cataloging in Publication Data

Jones, Peter, 1934–
    Swimming pools.

    1. Swimming pools. 2. Baths, Hot.   I. Title.
TH4763.J64   690′.89
AACR2
ISBN: 0-385-17280-X

Library of Congress Catalog Card Number
    81–43268

CONTENTS

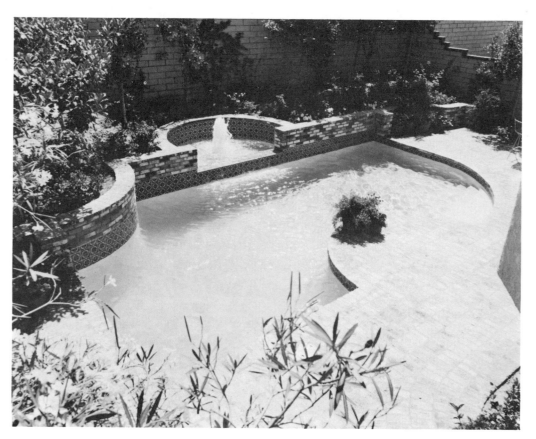

The only real reason anybody has a swimming pool is for the pure pleasure of their time splashing around in the water.

CHAPTER ONE

Why Have a Pool or Hot Tub?

Pleasure. When all is said and done, the only real reason that anyone would ever consider owning and maintaining a swimming pool or hot tub is the pure, unadulterated pleasure of splashing around in water. Psychologists can give you all kinds of sage observations about the early delights you experienced as a baby and then as a child splashing around in water, and how it soothed you, brought you relaxation. The philosophers can surely build a rationalization about your relationship with water, whether it is cold or warm, and describe it as a life-giving force that revitalizes the human body. The astrologers, psychics, and theologians can find a multitude of attachments between the human body and the soul and God as He is manifested in water. But when everybody gets finished with his considerations and estimations and explanations, the result is that splashing around in water just plain feels good. It feels so good that many people want that water available to them all or most of the time, so they dig a hole in the ground next to their homes and fill it with water.

Last year over 100,000 people spent anywhere from $5,000 to $15,000 installing a swimming pool in or on their private property. At the same time some 85,000 spas and hot tubs were also installed, so considering that those installation numbers continue to grow each year, it can be said that a considerable portion of the American population is in the process of doing something about the common human interest in spending part of the time submerged in water.

There are, of course, all sorts of rationales for spending several thousand dollars to possess a pool of water created solely for your private use. In some parts of the country, a swimming pool or hot tub or spa becomes an investment because it increases the value of real estate property. This is not, by the way, necessarily true in every state of the Union. The real value that a property is increased by is not an accounting or real estate function, but is based on common agreement in the specific locale.

Nevertheless, pools and hot tubs continue to be placed throughout the United States to the degree that there are now some two million private pools in America and their ranks are swelling by as much as 10 percent every year. It should be noted that even an economic recession does not slow down pool and hot tub sales very much. To begin with, family incomes continue to keep pace with inflation and more people than ever before are earning an income, with the result that both family and disposable incomes continue to rise. Moreover, as the petroleum shortage continues on again, off again, more and more people reduce their unnecessary traveling and this in turn creates the need for a family recreation center near home. About as close to home as you can get is your own back yard, so why not put a pool or hot tub in it? And as mortgage interest rates continue to rise, there are fewer and fewer housing starts so more and more homeowners are opting to remain where they are and extend their living quarters. For many, that extension includes adding a swimming pool and/or hot tub or spa.

THE COST OF INSTALLATION

In those parts of the country where a pool or hot tub is considered a property improvement, it is a sound long-term investment. Experts estimate that a good in-ground pool will endure for fifty or more years, which means that its cost is depreciating at something around 2 percent annually. Plus the fact that the presence of a pool in your yard will probably contribute to fewer vacations away from home, which, of course, cost money. But there are still parameters concerning the size and cost of the pool you install.

Real estate experts reckon that a swimming pool should not exceed more than 15 to 18 percent of the total value of your property. Thus, if you own a house and property worth $100,000, your swimming pool should not cost more than $18,000. By spending more than that, you will have trouble recouping your investment.

You are faced with installation costs of $5,000 and up for an honest-to-goodness pool that represents a permanent improvement to your property, and anywhere from $1,500 and up to install a hot tub or spa. Banks, federal savings and loan associations are, in most cases, able and willing to provide pool installation capital. If your present mortgage allows, you may be able to increase its balance by the amount needed to buy and install a pool or hot tub. Alternatively, you may be able to qualify for a home improvement loan and include the pool cost in that. And when all else fails, your local pool contractor or dealer can usually help to arrange financing either directly or as your representative with one of the lending institutions.

THE COST OF MAINTENANCE

An average-sized residential pool can cost anywhere from $25 to $50 a month to maintain, depending on the cost of chemicals to sanitize the water, the water itself, and the local rate for electricity to run the pump/filter and, if you have

one, the heater. The cost can be much higher if you employ someone to do the cleaning, sterilizing, and other chores that are a part of maintaining the pool and its water in clean, usable condition. Pool maintenance companies charge anywhere from $50 to $100 a month to do all of the dirty work of keeping your pool clean.

The trend in pool building has also given rise to a replacement and after market. Pools sometimes must be heated; the water in them must always be pumped through a filter system to keep it clean. The electric motors and pumps used to control pool water tend to need motor repairs after an average of seven years of use. Pool heaters will typically need replacement after about ten years. Then there are the cleaning equipment, diving boards, ladders, and accessories, plus the chemicals; and the after market in pools accounts for well over $500 million for just the major pool equipment, plus tens of millions of dollars for accessories after that. Don't get the notion that once you have financed and paid for your new swimming pool or hot tub that there are no more costs to be met. In some ways, the real expense begins when you fill the unit for the first time. Even so, you are likely to be spending less and getting more enjoyment than you would by taking vacations away from home every year.

AT THE BOTTOM OF POOLS

When the costs have been estimated and the decision is made to install a pool in your back yard, one fact remains. No matter how much it costs (providing its expense is within your budget), it will provide you and your family with hours of relatively inexpensive pleasure and relaxation. It will always be there for you to use as you step out of bed in the morning or before retiring at night, and any other time during the day or night. You will not have to get in your car and sit in barely moving beach traffic, or hunt for a parking space in the country club parking lot. It can be heated so that instead of using it two or three months of the year, you can enjoy your swimming all year long, depending, of course, on where you live. You can make your own rules and regulations about when to use your pool, and you can go swimming without being crowded out of the water. Best of all, it is yours. You own it. You care for it. In all probability, that gives you the right to enjoy it most of all.

CHAPTER TWO

Residential Swimming Pools

There are pneumatically applied concrete, poured concrete, vinyl liner in-ground, vinyl liner on-ground, and a host of other types of residential swimming pools. They can be round, oblong, or practically any shape you can imagine. Therein lies an inherent difficulty. Because pool shapes and sizes are unlimited, you can have anything that suits your space and your purposes, but determining exactly what it is that meets your needs can become a perplexing problem.

As you settle on a particular pool, you must consider its size, shape, and location, the type of structure, its trim, inside finish, color, the proper depths for swimming, wading, and diving, and the kind of equipment you want. You must also consider whether or not you possess the proper skills and can devote the time to building your own pool. In any case you will need, most likely, at least the services of an architect or engineer to help you settle on the kind of construction that is best suited for your climate and site. Your alternative is to hire a pool contractor, who not only has the equipment and knowledge to do the job for you, but probably also has a pool architect or engineer on his staff who can take care of such details as the pool plans.

YOUR POOL AND THE LAW

Before you get much further than the original urge to own a pool, check your local building code to be sure you are permitted to have a swimming pool on your property. In most locales you will need a building permit, and it is best to check your local zoning regulations and building codes to determine any special restrictions or requirements governing swimming pools. The requirements vary considerably from municipality to municipality and the only way you can know what they are is to consult your local building department. For example, some locales require only that there be a fence around any swimming pool. Others demand that filters can be installed only by a licensed plumber.

Usually, the installation will then have to be inspected at various points during its construction. Never begin any construction until all of the required permits have been issued (there will be one for the masonry, another for the plumbing, and at least a third for the electricity) or you are liable to be faced with some changes that could become costly.

Also take a look at your property deed restrictions. This will include setbacks from your property lines, permissible buildings, and easements of record for power or telephone cables, sewers and storm drains. Remember that as the property owner it is your responsibility to comply with the deed instructions; it is not the responsibility of any contractor or municipal department.

Finally, read the fine print in your homeowner's liability policy. Legally, a swimming pool is defined as an "attractive nuisance." In other words, if anyone falls into it and is hurt, you are liable, so make certain that your insurance is broad enough to protect you.

POOL SIZES

There is a notion that the bigger the pool, the more fun you can have, but that is not necessarily true. If it is properly designed and constructed, you can get plenty of enjoyment out of a 10' × 25' pool—and share that fun with a score of friends at the same time. In general, pools divide into three size categories: 15' × 30', 15' × 30' to 20' × 40', and 800 square feet (20' × 40') or larger. About 75 percent of all residential pools installed fit into the 15' × 30' to 20' × 40' category, but the size you install depends on a whole pile of factors.

Obviously, the smaller a pool, the less it costs, but the two criteria that most dictate pool size are: 1) the dimensions of the available land and 2) the number of people who will be using the pool. After you have considered those two factors, you also want to look at the size of your pool in relation to the size of the house and property. It would look a little ridiculous to have a 1,500-square-foot pool behind a two-room shack.

The walkways around the pool should be a minimum of 3' on all sides with a wider area of pavement surrounding the back of any diving boards or slides. If you have a standard diving board that is 12' long, it will extend approximately 9' behind the deep end of the pool. There should then be at least a 2' wide walking space behind the back end of the board. Consequently, if you install a 15' × 30' pool, with 3' walks and a 12' diving board, you will need an area measuring at least 21' × 44'. Beyond this minimum space requirement, you should allow enough room for plantings and/or fences. As a rule of thumb, you want to keep the pool at least 5'

from the nearest structure, whether it is a walkway, a fence, or a building.

Given ample space and adequate financial resources for whatever size pool you might want to install, the question becomes, "How big a pool do I need?" There is no iron-clad answer, but the rule most often applied is 36 square feet of water area for each swimmer, and 100 square feet for each diver. A 15' × 30' pool will provide 450 square feet of water surface. Divide by 36 square feet per swimmer and the pool can accommodate 12½ people at one time. Allowing 100 square feet of water surface around the diving board, the board can be in use and the pool will still permit 10 swimmers to have all of the water space they need.

Even with the several computations you can apply to determining the appropriate size of your swimming pool, perhaps the most important factor has no number that can be inserted in the formula. You must estimate whether the majority of people who will regularly be using the pool require water that is deep enough for wading, or swimming, or diving. If there are young children who have not yet learned to swim, it may be desirable to install a small wading pool near the main pool that is no more than 18" to 24" deep. Otherwise, your pool should have between 3' and 5' of shallow water and then fall off to a depth of between 8' and 8½' at the diving-board end of the pool.

THE GRAPH PAPER APPROACH

One way of plotting the location of a swimming pool is to map out your property on graph paper. To this end, you are likely to have among the papers pertaining to your home a survey map which outlines your property (with measurements) and the position of your home on its plot. You can use the survey map to translate an accurate picture of your property to a sheet of ruled graph paper. Or you can go outside and take measurements and construct your own survey map. In either case, the map as it is drawn on your graph paper should include measurements as well as the position of walks, patios, the house, trees, sewer and power lines, and all outbuildings. When you have located all obstacles on your map, you can begin to consider logical areas that might support your pool.

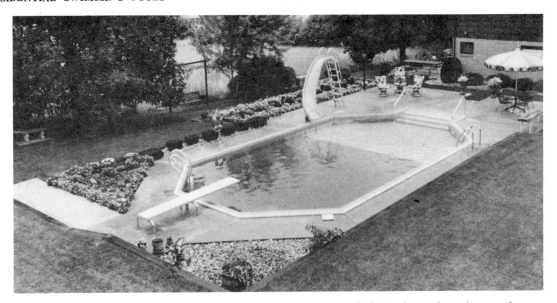

Diving boards and slides should have more walk area behind them than the usual 3′ that surrounds the pool.

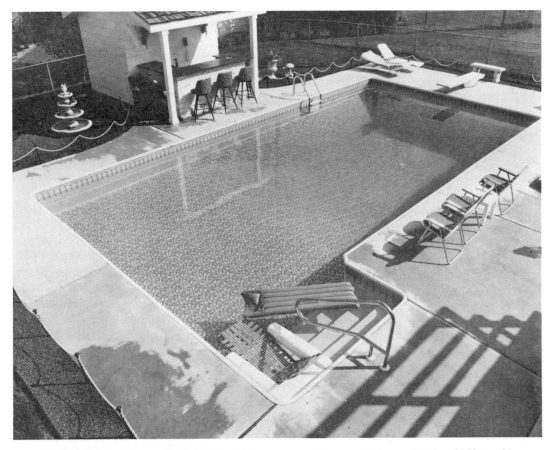

The bottom of a pool built for diving curves downward to a depth of 7′ to 9′ under the diving board.

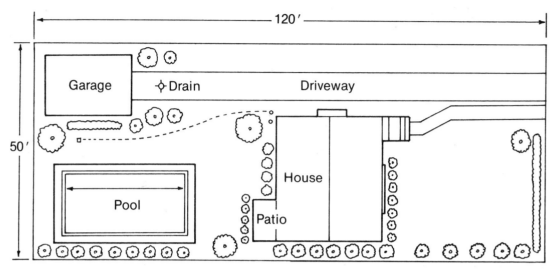

The most accurate way of plotting the exact position of your planned swimming pool is to measure your property and position every structure and plant on a sheet of graph paper.

LOCATING YOUR POOL

While it is quite acceptable to place your pool in an isolated recreational area of its own that may be well away from your house, most people put their pools as close to their homes as they can get them. Pools are most often placed in or next to a patio, or in a garden, or near a doorway that makes them easily accessible from the back or side of the building. Initially, determining exactly where you want to put your pool does not present any great problems. After you have done this, however, you have to make certain the area meets certain criteria, including some things that should *not* be present in the building site:

1. Either newly- or old-filled ground that is deeper than 3′ presents some costly structural changes that should be avoided. The pool must rest on solid soil, so make some test borings with a post-hole digger or by driving lengths of pipe into the ground to see what kind of earth you are dealing with.

2. The opposite extreme to filled ground is rock. If you decide to put your pool in a rocky area, be prepared for the added high expense of hiring pneumatic hammers and bulky removal equipment to gouge out and dispose of the rock. Your test borings will tell you soon enough if you are going to encounter solid rock formations,

and if that is what you discover, find some other place to put your pool. It is, of course, possible to partially bury a pool and rest it on a flat layer of rock that may be only a few feet below grade level. In this instance, you will have to do some building aboveground, but that is considerably cheaper and easier than hammering your way 10′ into bedrock.

3. Be very careful about underground springs or a water table that is close to the surface, causing soggy earth. Too much ground water, or soil that is mushy much of the time, indicates that you may have poor drainage or a high water table that will present some expensive problems during construction of the pool and conceivably will cause the pool to "float" after it is finished. If it does float, pressure against its underside from water rising up in the ground may cause the unit to break apart.

4. Make very certain there are no underground obstacles in the building site. A 300-gallon oil tank buried in your yard right where you decide to put your pool is going to be more trouble and expense to move than it is worth. But you also have to choose a site that is free of gas, sewer and drainage lines, or you might encounter telephone conduits, electrical feeder cables, old septic tanks or cesspools, buried walls, or filled-in basements or walls. If, by the way, you use a septic tank, your swimming pool must be placed a

minimum of 40′ away from it, as well as the sewage drain fields.

5. Try to avoid putting your pool in a steep slope. It might be nifty to look at when you get all finished, but to install it you are in for some heavy expenses for earth moving and for building retaining walls on the downhill side of the pool. If the site slopes only moderately, excavation can usually overcome the configuration of the land. If there are any questions in your mind about the true slope of your property, have a land survey made by a licensed surveyor. It should be noted that the same surveyor can also settle any questions you might have pertaining to the true location of your boundary lines.

6. It is long, tedious, and therefore expensive, to hand-move the amount of earth that must be removed to contain an in-ground swimming pool. Consequently, you should have an access avenue to the building site that is at least 8′ wide and 7′ or 8′ high so that earth-moving equipment

(trucks, backhoes, earthmovers) can be brought into the building site. If your property is small, the soil will have to be taken away from your premises. If you have a large plot, you might save a considerable amount of money by using the removed earth to landscape some other part of your property. Bear in mind that a 20′ × 40′ swimming pool will take up about 5,000 cubic feet, and that is a rather large mound of dirt to contend with, no matter what you do with it.

SOME ADVANCE PLANNING

Your pool ultimately will not stand unattached to the world around it, but must be linked to electrical, water supply, and water disposal systems. As you select the exact site for your pool, take the utilities into consideration:

1. There must be access to a fresh water supply line. Typically, the pool water comes from a ¾″ or 1″ hose bib extending from the side of

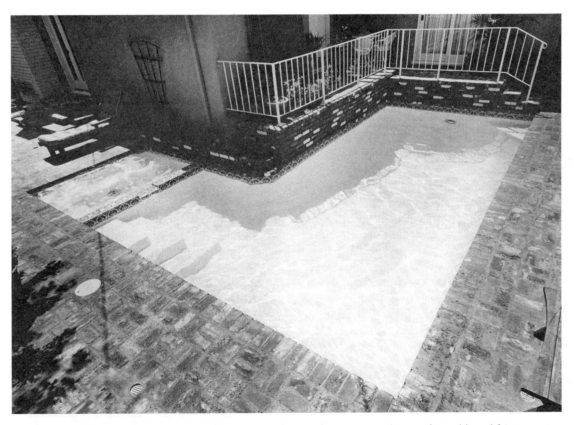

It would be hard to get a swimming pool any closer to the house than this, without putting it indoors.

your house, since it must have no connection whatsoever with the pool filter or the rest of the recirculating system. Bear in mind that if your pool does not have proximity to a water supply line you will need added pumping equipment to step up the normal 45 to 60 psi (pounds per square inch) of pressure in your house water supply system. Such equipment will markedly increase the cost of installation as well as operation of the pool.

2. Underwater pool lights, electricity to run the filter pump, and the heater controls (if you have a heater) must also be allowed for. Pool lights require a 110-volt circuit with the switch for the lights normally located in the house, rather than at the filter location or the pool itself. Most building codes call for a separate 110/220-volt circuit to handle the ½ to 1½ hp motors needed to operate pool pumps. Both circuits, because they are in proximity to water, must be protected by a Ground Fault Circuit Interrupter (GFCI). GFCI's are an expensive, but lifesaving device that will trip the circuit it protects and close off all electricity within 1/40 of a second, should there be even the hint of a short circuit. The rapid reaction of GFCI's will turn a potentially death-dealing electrical shock into a mild jolt, so they really are worth the extra cost.

3. You will have to plan for a backwash disposal system for the water used in the backwashing of certain types of sand filters. Essentially, part of the water in the pool is pumped through the filter, then forced back through the filter to cleanse it of all debris. The backwashing process is performed roughly every two weeks and requires between 300 and 800 gallons of water which cannot be returned to the pool, but must be disposed of. In some areas you can expel the used water into a municipal sewer system or storm drain. Elsewhere, you may need to dig a dry well to contain the water so that it can seep gradually into the ground. The water can also be used for irrigation and watering your grass, so long as you do not attach the filter backwash line to any small diameter hose that will restrict the flow of water and inhibit the proper backwash action.

4. If you intend to include a heater in your pool equipment, both the plumbing and heater's source of fuel must be considered. The diameter of the plumbing lines will depend on the individ-

ual unit and the heater capacity, and must also conform to your local plumbing code.

5. If you have impermeable or slow-draining soil, the floor of the pool can be placed on a 4″ to 6″ bed of sand, gravel, or crushed stone so that water outside the pool has a place to go. Alternatively, you can place a drain system around the base of the pool and connect it to a municipal sewer line, dry well, or storm drain.

The draining of surface water also requires some planning. Prior to any excavation, establish the elevation of the pool deck and slope it away from the pool so that no surface water can drain into the pool, but will run off to a lower ground level.

FINAL CONSIDERATIONS

Aside from having your pool in full view of your house and making it easily accessible and pleasant to look at, it should be situated to receive a maximum amount of sunlight each day. But while the sun's rays are desirable, the prevailing breezes that habitually play across your property can cause more problems than they are worth. The wind will, among other things, cool the water and make it evaporate, making swimming uncomfortable. People usually block off the wind either with fences or windscreens, or shrubbery. These same fences and shrubbery can also be used to provide a measure of privacy around the pool and help to discourage children and adults alike from wandering into the pool uninvited.

If you build your pool and do not provide separate dressing room facilities, the pool should be close enough to the house to permit convenient changing. It is also customary to place the shallow end of the pool nearest the house so that guests stepping out of the house and falling unawares into the pool don't find themselves thrashing around in deep water when they thought they were just going for a stroll in the garden.

To this same point, the diving board should be placed at the south or west end of the pool to prevent divers from being blinded by the sunlight. And trees and shrubbery that might deposit leaves, blossoms, or branches in the water should be kept well away from the pool swimming area —unless you want to spend an inordinate amount of leisure time fishing debris out of your pool.

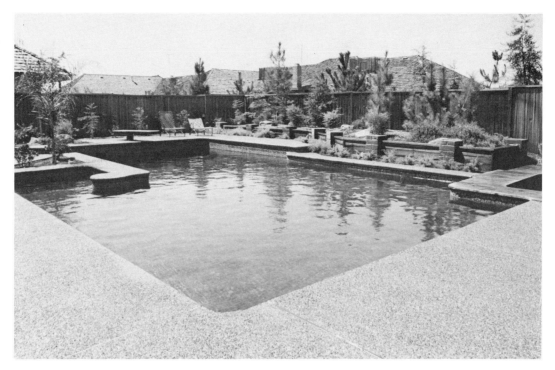

Pool owners usually try to block off the wind by erecting fences and planting shrubbery.

POOL SHAPES

Once you have selected a site for your pool, the next question usually concerns its shape. The answer is usually dependent on the architecture of your house, the design of your garden and the grounds around it, plus your personal preference. Here is a summary of the advantages of different pool shapes:

RECTANGLE

The standard rectangular pool, which is twice as long as it is wide, is considered the most utility oriented of all the pool shapes. It offers a maximum amount of swimming and diving space for the money you have to spend, and it looks particularly well when surrounded by relatively flat grounds. The way you get individuality and beauty out of a rectangular hole in the ground is by making the most out of the surrounding walks and landscaping. Color is added by the paints you use on the pool, as well as the kind of pool equipment and its color. Rectangular pools will go well with any architectural design.

OVAL

An oval pool will also go well with any architectural style and can reside in practically any location. You can do some magnificent decorating around an oval pool, so it is considered to be the most beautiful of all the pool shapes. What you gain in magnificence, however, is somewhat lost in utility. The rounded ends restrict the swimming and diving areas somewhat in comparison with the rectangle.

KIDNEY AND MOUNTAIN LAKE

The kidney shape is often used with hillside homes having irregular terrain. If those irregularities are moderate, the kidney shape can usually be worked around the varying ground levels. If the grounds vary greatly, the most practical approach is a free-form version of the kidney shape known as the mountain lake. The mountain lake still has a squeezed portion but the rest of the kidney shape may be stretched out of symmetry to accommodate the terrain. It goes without saying that swimming becomes somewhat re-

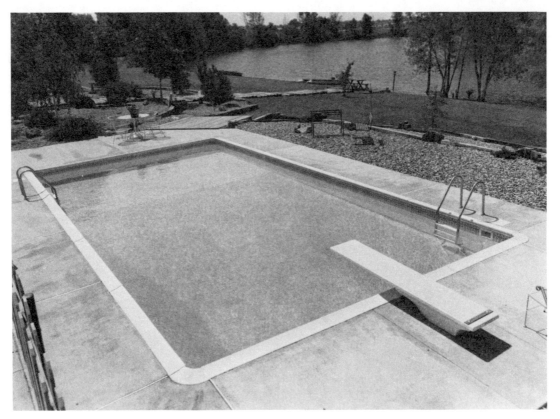

The rectangular shape.

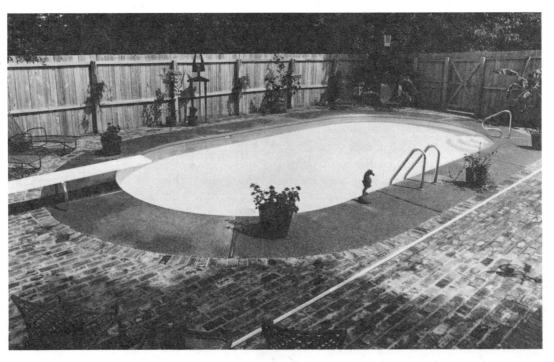

The oval.

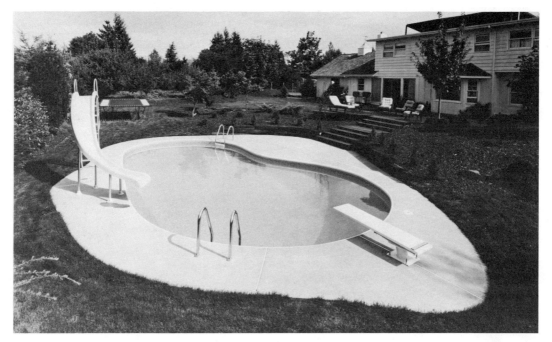

The kidney shape.

stricted but the inherent beauty of a pool fitted into the existing terrain is unparalleled.

FREE-FORM

When the terrain is really difficult to fit a pool into, the usual solution is a free-form pool. This can be any shape or size dictated by the land formations, and because it is free-form you have the opportunity of taking full advantage of the sun as well as shaded and protected areas and the view, plus gaining all the privacy you may wish to have. You do all this, of course, by manipulating terraces, patios, walkways, trees, and shrubbery and then shaping the pool to fit into whatever space you have left.

It should be noted that while a rectangular pool will probably give you the best cost per square foot, a custom-built swimming pool that takes up every inch of usable space and offers a unique aesthetic quality to your property will not cost a great deal more than plunking down a standard-shaped pool of comparable dimensions.

POOL TYPES

A *residential swimming pool* is defined by the swimming pool industry as "any constructed pool, permanent or portable, which is intended for noncommercial use as a swimming pool by not more than three owner families and their guests, and which is more than 24″ deep and has either a surface area exceeding 250 square feet, or a volume of more than 3,250 gallons." There are five types of residential pool classifications, divided according to their suitability for different types of diving equipment. Type I is any residential pool where the installation of diving equipment is prohibited. Type II through Type V are suitable for different kinds of diving equipment.

Swimming pools are further defined according to the type of structure:

Permanently Installed Swimming Pools are constructed in the ground or in a building in such a way that they cannot readily be dismantled.

Nonpermanently Installed Swimming Pools are constructed so they can be easily disassembled and then be put back together again to their original integrity.

In-ground Swimming Pools have their sides resting partially or wholly in contact with the surrounding earth.

On-ground Swimming Pools have sides that are fully above the ground.

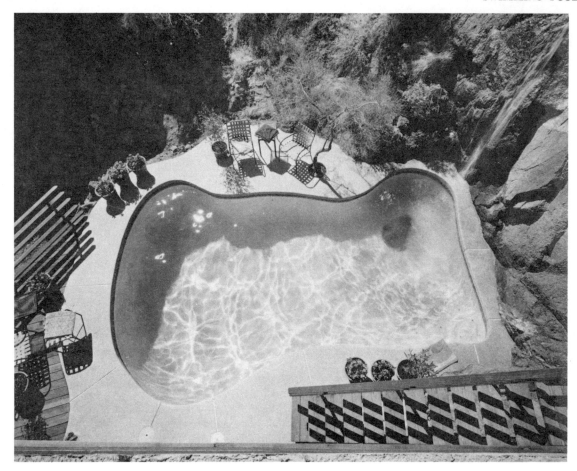

The free-form.

Aboveground/Portable Pools are removable. They can be any shape but must be more than 42″ deep or hold more than 2,500 gallons, or have a water surface of 150 or more square feet. The frame of an aboveground pool must be entirely above grade level, and be readily disassembled and reassembled to its original integrity.

Wading Pools can be any shape or size and have a depth of from zero to 3′. It is hard to swim in 3′ of water, so wading pools are specifically to be used for wading.

Just for the record, public pools are any pools other than residential pools and come in four classifications (A, B, C, and D) as well as types VI through IX. By definition, a public pool is "intended for swimming or bathing and is operated by an owner or leasee, operator licensee, or concessionaire, regardless of whether a fee is charged for use."

POOL CONSTRUCTION

About 54 percent of all the pools built in America are made of pneumatically applied concrete. A little over 4 percent are poured concrete construction and 34 percent have vinyl liners. The remaining 8 percent or so are made of fiberglass, metal, and other materials. All of these pools, no matter what their construction, are built to a long list of minimum standards that are suggested by the National Swimming Pool Institute to ensure that every residential pool meets minimal safety standards and good workmanship.

PNEUMATICALLY APPLIED CONCRETE

The most popular method for building a residential pool is pneumatically applied concrete, known as *Gunite*. The great advantage of Gunite is that it can be easily shaped into any form desired; the disadvantage is its slightly higher cost.

The Gunite construction process is relatively simple and much quicker than other forms of concrete construction. The excavation is dug to the exact shape of the finished pool and is then lined with steel reinforcing rods that are placed in a gridwork along the sides and bottom of the excavation. The Gunite is a mixture of hydrated cement and sand in a semi-liquid state which is applied over, under, and around the metal rods under air pressure. The Gunite comes from a transit mixer and is fired through a pressure nozzle that permits it to be laid to the proper thickness to ensure against air pockets and prevent any areas of loose sand. You have to have all of your plumbing lines in place before any of the Gunite is applied, and all inlets and outlets must be covered with plastic so they do not become clogged by the concrete.

Gunite has a rough texture and must be trimmed by hand before a finish coat of plaster or paint is applied over it. However, as soon as the Gunite is in place, the finishers can move in to trim the walls and floor of the pool and cut skimmer and other openings necessary to make the pool functional.

POURED CONCRETE

While poured concrete is not used for more than 5 percent of the pools built today, it is still an approved method of constructing a residential swimming pool. The concrete can be poured into forms, used in conjunction with concrete blocks, or hand-packed without the use of any forms whatsoever.

With the traditional poured concrete method, the excavation is lined with wooden forms that are then filled with cement. The use of forms requires a considerable amount of labor, particularly in pools that contain curves of any sort, so poured concrete pools tend to be rectangular and have more or less vertical walls.

A somewhat simpler method of applying poured concrete is first to excavate the pool site and then pour concrete over reinforcing rods laid over the floor of the pool. Specially grooved concrete blocks are then stacked around the perimeter of the floor but are not mortared together. The blocks are stood over reinforcing rods that have been anchored to the concrete floor plate

and are threaded at their tops. Cement is then poured into the blocks, producing a solid concrete wall and wall-top plates are bolted to the threaded tops of the reinforcing rods. The inside of the pool is then coated with cement which is troweled on the blocks to a thickness of 1″ to 1½″.

Still another method of construction is known as hand-packed concrete. Basically, the concrete is mixed with less moisture and sometimes has a bonding agent blended into it. It is then placed by hand around reinforcing rods. In order to keep the concrete in place, the walls must slope and both the corners of the pool as well as the joint where the floor and walls meet are usually curved.

VINYL LINER CONSTRUCTION

Pools having liners are normally aboveground or portable designs. The shell of the pool may be concrete blocks, poured concrete, or some other rigid material that need not be waterproof, only sturdy. The vinyl liner is a sealed membrane that provides a watertight envelope that is installed in any manner that will protect it from slipping around inside its shell.

FIBERGLASS CONSTRUCTION

Fiberglass pool shells are delivered to the pool site in one big shell and placed in the excavation or between sturdy walls. They can be molded to any shape or size and provide a durable, smooth surface for the pool, but they tend to be expensive.

WALL AND FLOOR CONFIGURATIONS

There are no limitations on the shape of a swimming pool except in terms of its safety and the recirculation of its water. There should not be, however, submerged protrusions, extensions, or anything that can entangle or obstruct a swimmer.

There are some recommendations by the National Swimming Pool Institute about pool depths and other design dimensions. Water depths, for instance, should be between 2′9″ and 3′6″ at the shallow end of the pool. The pool walls at the shallow end should be vertical from the water line down at least 2′3″. From that

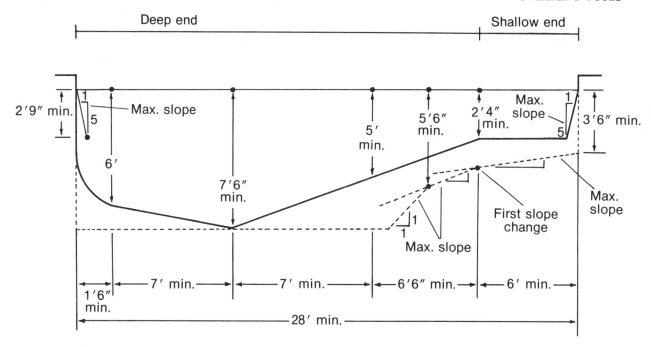

Anatomy of the minimum dimensions of a pool designed for diving.

point the wall can curve to meet the pool floor. The floor in most pools slopes toward the deep end and this slope should be no more than 1′ of drop for every 7 linear feet, to the point of the first slope change. The Pool Institute defines the point of the first slope change as, "the point at which the floor slope exceeds one foot (1′) in seven feet (7′), and is at least six feet (6′) from the shallow end wall."

The point of the first slope change is the beginning of a steeper slope that is recommended to be 1′ in every 2′6″. This slope continues to a point where the depth of the water is 5′6″. From that depth to the deep end of the pool, the floor slope is not to exceed 1′ for every foot of its run.

A depth of 5′ or 6′ is quite enough for swimming in flat-bottom pools that are restricted from incorporating diving equipment. Pools designed to be used with diving equipment are another animal. If you install an 8′ or 10′ diving board, placed close to the pool deck, the deep end of the pool can be as shallow as 7′. The recommended depth is 8′ with a 10′ diving board positioned 18″ above the surface of the water. If the diving board is a regulation one meter board, it should be 39.37″ above the water which should have a depth of at least 8′6″. The minimum

allowable depth should be extended at least 4′ beyond the end of the board and the slope of the pool bottom may be steep directly under the board, that is at the deep end of the pool. Note the following chart, which not only shows the minimum depths for different boards, but also the recommended distances from the side walls to the board overhang.

POOL TRIM

The trim surrounding a pool includes the walkway, decking, and coping, which resides around the top of the pool walls, the way molding is placed around a window or doorframe. All three elements must be evaluated from both an aesthetic and an economic point of view. In other words, you need to consider a variety of materials and designs and choose those that are compatible with the over-all décor surrounding the pool; then you have to make certain you can afford the particular materials you have selected.

WALKS AND DECKING

The walkway around your pool should be nonabsorbent and slip proof, as well as easily cleanable. You can use brick, flagstone, or brushed concrete

DIVING AREA

MINIMUM DEPTHS AND AREAS

Boards	Max. Distance Above Water	Min. Overhang	Distance from Diving Wall	Min. Width to Each Side of Board	Min. Depth
Deck Level	18″	2′	10′	7′	7′
Residential	28″	2½′	11′	7½′	8′
1 Meter	39.37″	3′	12′	9′	9′

that has a color pigment added to it when it is mixed, or merely painted. Actually you can use just about any material that can withstand constant weathering but the brushed concrete is most likely the least expensive, unless you live near a brick factory or rock quarry. It is important when laying any decking that the area be sloped a minimum of ¼″ for every running foot *away* from the pool, to prevent runoff from getting into the bathing water.

With block or poured concrete pools, be careful that the backfill (the earth replaced in the hole behind the forms) has had ample time to settle, which could mean as long as six months before any decking is laid. The walks should be a minimum of 3′ wide, and if you have the space you might consider a larger area at the shallow end of the pool or along one side that can be paved to permit sun-bathing, eating, and other activities. This will tend to keep some of the people enjoying the pool out of the water and reduce the number of swimmers and divers in the pool at one time, with the result that your pool will have a greater capacity and tend to remain cleaner for longer periods of time.

COPING AND TILE

The coping around the top of the pool walls is, on the average, 12″ to 15″ wide. Its purpose is to enhance the looks of the pool and normally it is made of precast stone with a single bull-nose, which provides a handhold as well as a raised lip that tends to shed runoff away from the pool. There are, of course, alternative materials that can be used for the coping, including tile, brick, metal, even some of the plastics.

Evaporation and use of the pool normally cause a variation in the water level from day to day. Consequently, the top 4″ to 6″ of pool walls

are often faced with a decorative tile which ends under the lip of the coping. If the area is subject to freezing temperatures, the tiles used must be full vitreous all-weather products. Otherwise, nearly any tile will suffice so long as it is installed according to the manufacturer's instructions. While the most usual color for the tiles is blue, you can actually use any of the warm colors, such as peach, maroon, or orange, since they will contrast with and intensify the blue color of the pool water.

INTERIOR POOL FINISHING

The final step in the construction of your pool will be to apply an interior finish to the bottom and walls, which normally has a color of some sort. So you have to consider what that color is to be in the planning stages of the pool. A proper interior finish should be light in color, watertight, smooth, easy to clean, and impervious to just about everything. The finish itself should not have any rough or uneven spots that can catch dirt and possibly cause skin abrasions. Consequently, the materials most often used to finish the interior of pools are paint, tile, or a kind of plaster made of silica sand, hard white marble, and a bonding agent. Strong, dark colors applied to the inside of pools are generally considered to create too harsh an effect. The choice is practically always in the blue family, usually a pale blue or turquoise. Actually, filtered water against a white finish causes the pool to look as though it were a brilliant blue, so it is really unnecessary to use any color in the pool finish itself. This is particularly true of the silica sand/white marble plaster, which produces a brilliant turquoise-blue color. The plaster, which is actually much harder than ordinary plaster, does not contain any lime, which would disintegrate under water, and is

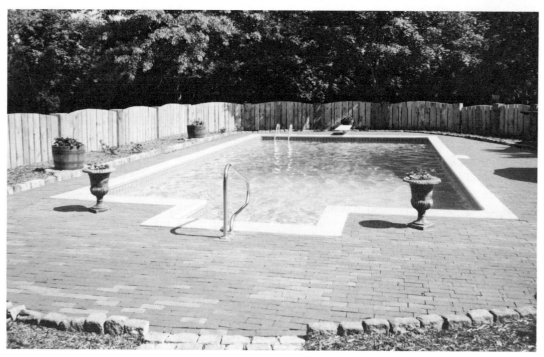

The decking around a pool can be made of any durable, weatherproof material, including wood, concrete, stone, or brick.

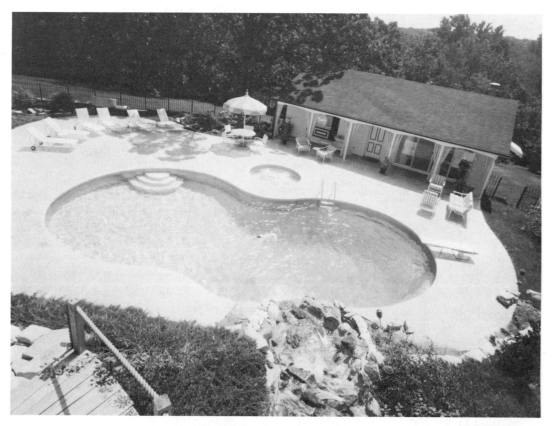

An extended area around the shallow end of the pool can be used for sun-bathing, partying, or any number of pool-related activities.

more impervious to damage than even the concrete shell of the pool. Fortunately, it is still the least expensive of all the finishes used on the interior of pools.

SPACE FOR THE FILTERS

The filter system that attends your pool, and is necessary for keeping the water clean and sanitary, must be allotted enough space near the pool for its installation. The filter is usually positioned at one end of the installation on a concrete slab that is within 20′ or 30′ of the pool itself. You can house the filter, its pump, and motor in a shed, a corner of your garage, against an inside corner of the house, even underground. You can also leave them out in the open, although in cold climates it is better to give them some sort of protection. So far as your planning is concerned, you need only choose a location for the filter and pump, and decide how to decorate it, whether it is with a flower bed, shrubbery, decking, or whatever. Since the filters and pumps are available in a wide variety of sizes and shapes, it is best to follow the manufacturer's specifications about the amount of space their installation requires.

ACCESSORIES

While you may not want to include all of the available swimming pool accessories at the time you build your pool, keep in the back of your mind that the day may come when you want to add some of them. Consider, then, allowing space for such things as a diving board, ladders, pool covers, chlorinators, life lines, and so forth, during your planning stage, even if you decide not to include them at the time of installation.

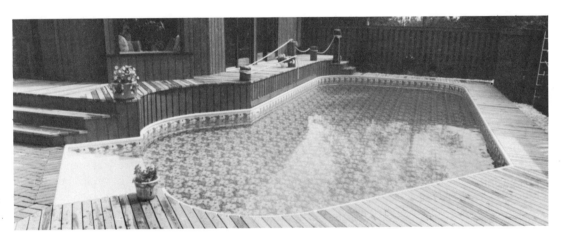

The interior of this pool was constructed of tiles, but it might have been any of several other durable materials.

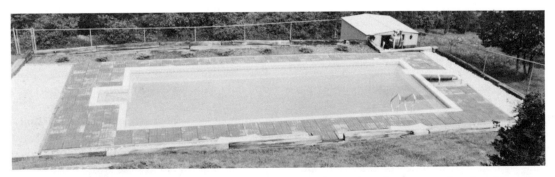

The filter system, pump, heater, and other accessories and equipment can be stored in their own building near the pool.

CHAPTER THREE

Ways of Building a Swimming Pool

People usually take one of three approaches when building a swimming pool. They 1) have it entirely constructed by a pool contractor, 2) have it partially built by professional labor and partially by themselves, or 3) buy a pool package and build it themselves.

PACKAGE POOLS

Before you undertake the installation of a large in-ground pool (over 15' × 30') you would be wise to develop a proficiency in such construction techniques as concrete and masonry work, earth removal, electricity, plumbing, and design. A pool that is 20' × 40' weighs about 150 tons when it is filled with water, which means you are dealing with some potent forces of stress and weight. Those forces are not reduced appreciably by a smaller-sized pool, so no matter what type of pool you elect to build yourself you are up against some complicated problems concerning reinforcement of the materials you use.

You can purchase in-ground as well as on-ground, aboveground, and portable pool packages and by doing all or much of the installation work yourself, you can cut your expenses in half. Pool packages contain everything, including a vinyl liner, vacuum cleaner, filter system, coping, skimmer box, fittings, even a starter chemical kit, and you can get them in just about any size you might want or need. All you have to do is follow the manufacturer's installation instruction sheet, which is even likely to give you some hints about the excavation that will have to be done first. The masonry work, if there is any needed, is likely to be left entirely up to you.

With all that construction information provided in a pool package, it is still a good idea to spend the few extra dollars for some professional consultation either with a pool architect or engineer, or perhaps your local pool dealer. There are too many personal preferences, building code limitations, and just plain details to consider for anybody to wing it at the cost of several thousand dollars and a considerable amount of your time and labor. You have to carefully plan out not only the pool itself, but also your electrical circuits, water supply, drainage and sewer, landscaping, and a host of minute details that may not appear evident at first glance.

If you are constructing an in-ground pool, your most formidable task is the excavation, and even if the pool is only a moderate size, digging a hole for it in your back yard demands an uncon-

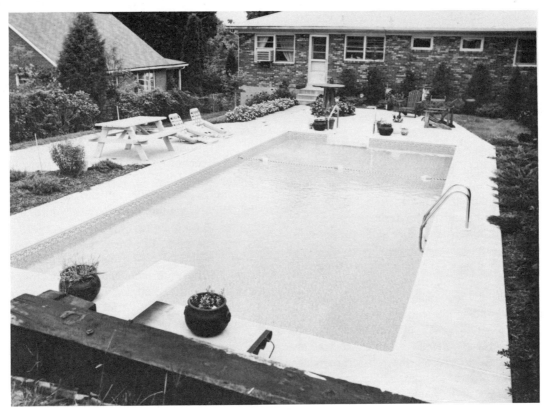

To install an in-ground pool on your own you should have a proficiency in a variety of construction techniques.

scionable amount of spade work. It is quicker and infinitely more efficient to hire a contractor to dig the hole and remove the earth (either off your premises or to some part of your property that needs regrading). The contractor will arrive with a backhoe or similar earth-moving equipment and probably require less than a day to do what could take you months working by hand.

Once the hole is dug, your next chore is to build the floor and walls of the pool and how you do that depends on the product you have purchased. The floor of the pool must be graded to the proper depths and concrete footings must be poured into trenches dug around the perimeter of the floor. If the floor is to be concrete, it is poured into wooden forms. Forms for the walls must also be constructed, unless they are to be made of concrete blocks. The blocks are laid up around ½″ reinforcing steel rods and the space between them and the sides of the excavation are backfilled with sand or gravel to provide a solid backing. The floor, if it is merely to support a

liner, can then be graded with sand. If you are using a liner, it is attached over the top of the walls and its hem is covered by the wall coping.

Some pool packages consist of a metal or fiberglass shell which is delivered to your excavation as a single unit ready to accept its plumbing and electrical connections. Other packages consist of steel or aluminum panels which are assembled either completely in the ground or only partially below grade. Obviously, if half of the pool stands aboveground, the excavation will not be as deep as a completely in-ground pool.

Aboveground/portable pools are designed to be assembled in your back yard and then disassembled whenever you want to store or move them. These units are often just stood up in your yard and people get in and out of them via a ladder. If any elevated decks are built around an on-ground pool, however, the platform must be provided with rails around the entire outside perimeter that are no less than 27″ high above the deck. Actually, the aboveground portable swimming pools sold today are required by the National Swimming Pool Institute to be protected by a fence, wall, or enclosure made of a durable material, and the gate leading through that enclosure must have a permanent means of locking that is inaccessible to small children from the outside.

DOING PART OF THE WORK YOURSELF

You can, without question, reduce the installation cost of any swimming pool by doing part of the work yourself. You can save considerably just by purchasing all the materials yourself and hiring a local mason and other subcontractors to do the work. By doing your own purchasing and contracting, you may save as much as 20 percent of the installation cost. But be sure you have a set of well-designed plans and that you are around the building site enough during the work process to assure yourself that all of the standards of safety and strength are met. If you are not very careful to oversee the job scrupulously, you could wind up spending 20 percent more than it would cost to have a contractor do the whole job. The work schedule you will have to follow is something like this:

Pool plans. To get a good set of plans, you need to hire an engineer or pool architect.

Permits. The plans for your pool and a copy of your site plan or a plot survey of your property must be taken to your local building department. The department will review the plans and issue permits for the masonry, plumbing, and electrical work. You could have the person who designed the plans get the permits for you, but you will be charged for his or her time.

Excavation of the pool. You could dig the hole in your yard by yourself, but it is more efficient and infinitely faster to hire a contractor who has a backhoe and a truck to dig the excavation and remove the excess earth.

Concrete work. For this, you need a mason unless you are experienced at mixing and placing concrete. You could have the forms built by a carpenter or build them yourself and then have the concrete delivered to your site already mixed. If you have never worked with concrete before, it is better to have a mason on hand.

Pool liner. This may entail tile work or applying hydrated cement and silica sand, both of which require a skill gained only from practice.

The mason should be qualified to handle the job. If the liner is plastic, install it on your own.

Backfilling. This you can do yourself, or if the job is too big, hire some day laborers. It entails pushing dirt into the spaces between the excavation and the pool walls and tamping it down solidly.

Installing the filter and plumbing. Plumbing is not a very complicated chore and given installation instructions from the manufacturer and a working knowledge of standard plumbing practices you could get through this stage with relatively little trouble. Alternatively, hire a local plumber to do the work.

Electrical work. Electricity is no more complicated than plumbing. But the standards and regulations set forth in the National Electric Code and by your local building department can make electrical work a little tricky. If you have any doubts, hire an electrician.

Deck and patio. Decks may need to be supported by piers, which in turn rest on concrete footings in the ground. So a mason is in order unless you have learned enough from the mason you hired to do the pool to make your own footings. Patios can be excavated and laid by an amateur, or you can have them done by a mason. The decks, if they are wooden, amount to laying a floor across joists (which are supported by the piers). It is basically a rough carpentry job that does not really need the services of a carpenter. If you decide to hire someone, you can use carpenters hired at a daily or per job rate, or a contractor.

Cleanup. When you get all finished, there will be mounds of debris all over your yard. You can borrow or rent a truck and remove it yourself. For not an awful lot of money you can hire a removal company to do the same job faster and easier.

HIRING A CONTRACTOR

By far the easiest, and the most expensive, way of getting any pool installed is to hire a pool contractor to put it in for you. When you hire a reputable contractor, you can get a guarantee with the job and because of that guarantee the job is likely to be overbuilt to protect his reputation. Reputable pool contractors cannot afford to have their products spring a leak or in any way be less than satisfactory, or the word will get around

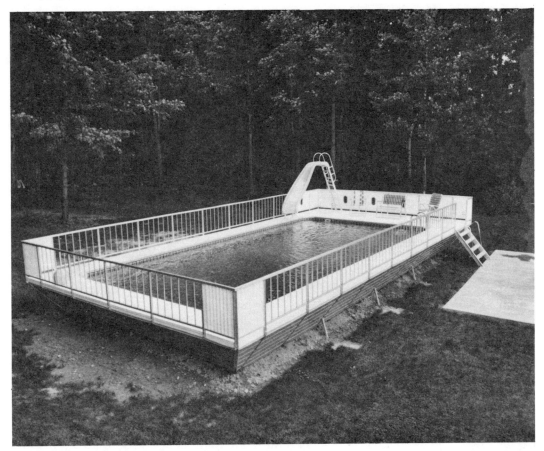

The excavation for a partially in-ground pool is not as deep as for one that is completely in-ground.

very quickly that they are not reputable contractors at all. Consequently, they will often make the pools they construct a little bit stronger at the expense of more time and materials (and more of your money). But the advantage is that you end up with a pool that demands less attention and is more durable.

A swimming pool can be constructed during almost any part of the year except in the coldest part of the winter in northern regions. But the time most people have their pools installed is the late spring through early fall. It is during that period that pool contractors everywhere are busiest and, because of the laws of supply and demand, their prices are also highest. One of the ways to reduce the cost of a swimming pool is to catch a contractor when he has little or nothing to do and is in a mood to take a lower profit just to have work for his men. He also has more time to

spend between the late fall and early spring, which means his attention is focused on what he is doing for you, and not on six or seven jobs going on at the same time. The result of that focused attention is that there are apt to be fewer mistakes made.

You also have a greater selection of pool contractors to pick from during the off season, but perhaps the best reason for building a pool in the winter is a technical one. Concrete (and Gunite) requires as much as a month of curing time in damp, cool conditions before the concrete reaches 100 percent of its strength. If you have built your pool in the late fall and it must then sit there exposed to winter weather for a couple of months, it will attain its optimum strength by early spring, when it can be painted and the landscaping around it can best be done. By that time you will have gotten used to having a pool in your yard and had time enough to completely design the way you want your yard to look.

POOL CONTRACTS

When you select a pool contractor, you are on the verge of handing over to him thousands of dollars in return for a specified pool that meets all of the standards of construction and safety. To protect both you and the contractor, there should be a full, written agreement that stipulates the nature and extent of *all* work to be done, as well as all of the costs of that work. Having a full contract that specifies every activity and cost to be undertaken may sound self-evident, but it is surprising how often people blithely pay out thousands of dollars to contractors without the slightest assurance in writing that they will be given a full measure of workmanship in return. There are some broad guidelines that you can

follow when selecting and hiring any contractor:

1. Pick a company that has a sound financial rating and a good reputation. You can ask for bank and customer references and call enough of them to be assured in your own mind that you are dealing with a reputable firm. If you are confident that the company you have selected is financially sound and professionally accepted, you have eliminated practically all of your worries.

2. The contract you are asked to sign should have no blank spaces in it and there are few reasons to have any extra charges, either. There should be a single, firm cost stated in the contract with no room for any surprises later on.

3. Know the name of the salesman you deal with and also know the name and address of the firm he represents.

4. Be sure that the salesman actually does rep-

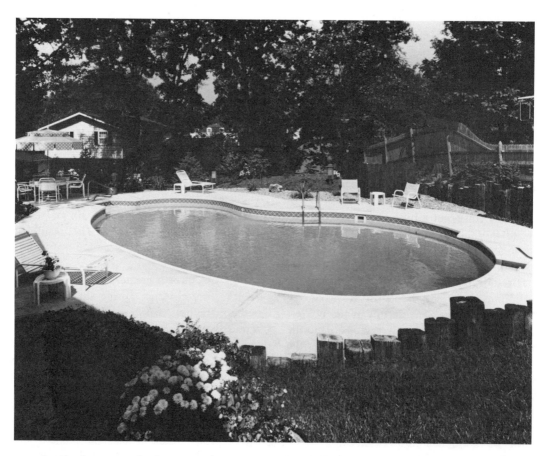

In the long run, having a pool contractor do all the installation work may be the least expensive way of getting your pool in place.

resent the firm he claims to represent.

5. All guarantees (for parts of, or the entire job) should be clearly stated in the contract. Make certain that the company will be able to fulfill those guarantees.

6. Be sure the company provides liability and compensation insurance for its workmen. If it does not, and one of its workmen is injured while working on your property, *you* are liable.

7. If the contractor is providing some or all the financing, there is a financing company lurking in the background somewhere. Know which company that is.

8. Never give anybody any cash. Even with a bill marked "paid" you have no sure record of what happens to the money. Pay everything with checks or money orders.

9. The contract should stipulate the time and place and to whom all payments are to be made.

10. If any part of the work is to be subcontracted for, the contract must protect you against liens on your home. This is usually done by the contractor's posting a completion bond or an escrow agreement, or with a lien release from each of the subcontractors.

11. Be certain the contract states that any damages occurring to your property during the construction work will be repaired at no cost to you.

12. The contract must state full specifications for the type and extent of work, when that work will be completed, the nature and cost of all extras, full descriptions of all materials (their quality, grade or name, weight, color, style) and the total cost including all financing charges.

13. All verbal representations made to you must be verified in the contract. Otherwise they might as well never have been made.

14. There should be a cancellation fee should you wish to terminate the contract at any time. Be sure all of your obligations are clearly stated.

15. Read and completely understand the entire contract before you sign it.

16. Be certain that the company officer who also signs the contract is a qualified member of the contracting firm.

Even with a fully defined contract in your hands, you may have some missing elements to look out for. There could be some additional charges for hooking up the gas lines and heater, as well as an additional expense (paid to your local power company) for bringing in more electrical lines.

And finally, do not sign any certificates of completion or turn over the last payment on the contract until *all* of the work is finished. The moment you let go of your final payment you have no "hook" in the contractor to come back and finish whatever small details may have been overlooked.

It is easy for any unscrupulous contractor to bilk you in a variety of ways. He can cheat on the quality of materials he uses, stint on the amount of labor he puts into the job, be shoddy about portions of the job that will be covered up by the ground, or decking, or any of the finishing materials. If he fails to pay his bills, liens can be placed on whatever property he is working on, forcing the property owner to pay for his pool twice, once to remove the liens and again to have the job completed by someone else. There are just too many ways to be cheated and you are involved in spending too much money not to give yourself a break by thoroughly investigating the company and people you are hiring, before you hire them. If you arrive at a proper contractual agreement with a reputable contractor who is an experienced pool builder, having your pool built can be a worry-free, relatively painless, and perhaps in the long run even less expensive experience than constructing your pool in any other manner.

BIRTH OF A GUNITE SWIMMING POOL

If you are thinking about saving some of the $15,000 it costs to have an in-ground swimming pool constructed for you, consider the specialized work and equipment you will need. Thumb through the next few pages and decide whether you are qualified to do the kind of work that must be done.

The swimming pool shown here was constructed for Mr. and Mrs. James Mazza by the St. G Pools, Inc., of Lambertville, New Jersey. St. G Pools builds forty to fifty pools every year using traveling crews of specialists who work in a four-state area (New York, Delaware, Pennsylvania, New Jersey). But it is St. G's reputation that is on the line, so the construction of every pool tends to be of inordinate quality.

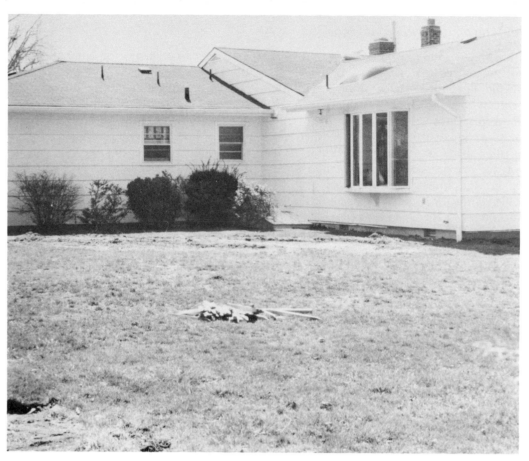

The Mazzas decided to place their pool with the diving end facing south, between the wings of their ranch-style house.

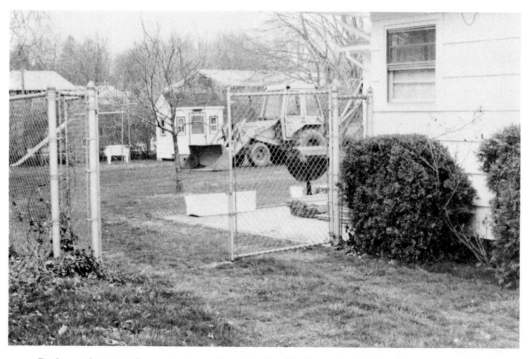

Perhaps the most important requirement for digging a pool is to have easy access to the construction site so that heavy machinery can reach it.

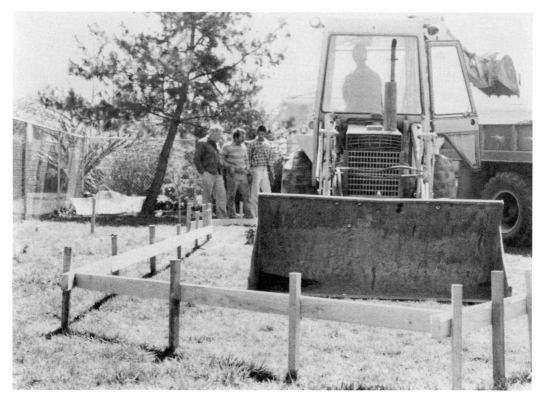

The outline of the pool must first be staked out and is precisely framed by 2″ × 4″'s leveled in all directions.

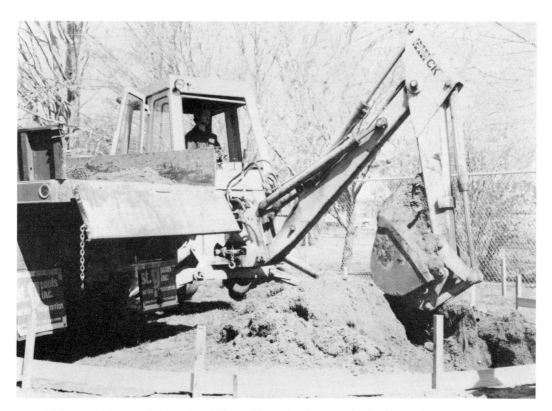

This particular pool is to be 18′ × 40′ and will contain 30,000 gallons of water—therefore about 45,000 cubic feet of earth must be carved out of the Mazzas' back yard and removed from the premises.

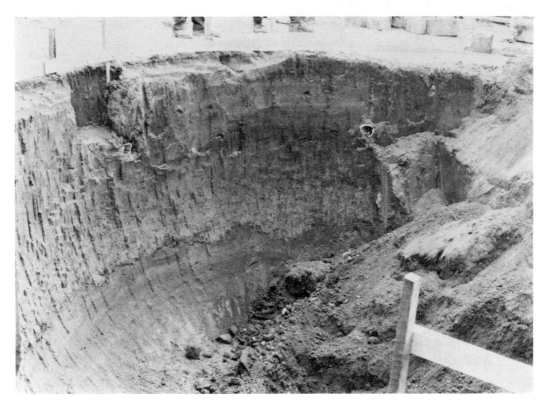

The deep end of the pool must go down some 8'6". Note the broken end of an old sewer pipe, which led to a septic tank. The notch in the edge of the excavation is for the underwater light.

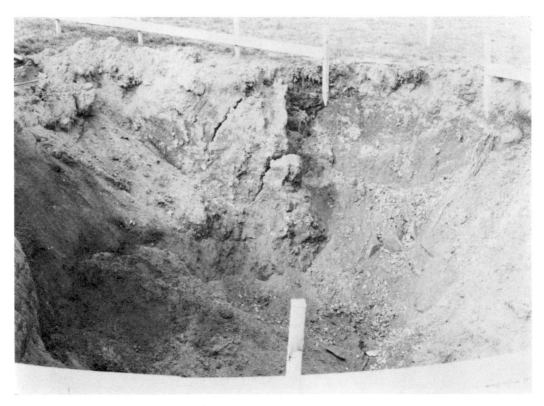

A complication arose when the diggers encountered the septic tank at the right side of the deep end of the pool. When the tank was removed, part of the excavation collapsed, leaving a hole that could not immediately be filled.

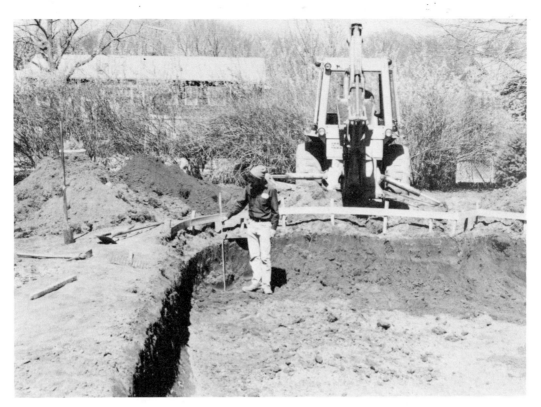

The bottom of the pool had to curve up to a level of 4'3″ in depth at the shallow end.

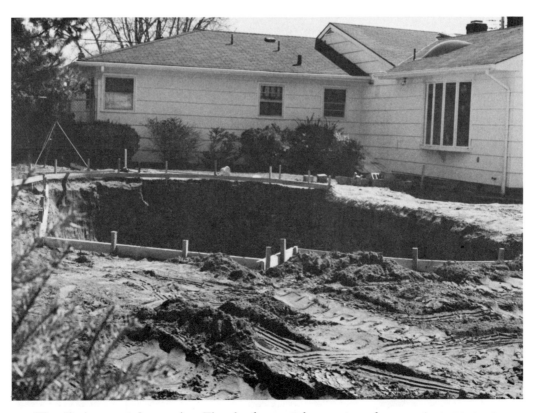

The digging must be precise. The depths must be exact, and so must every curve. Given two deep-bed dump trucks and a backhoe, a pool of this size is normally dug in less than a day.

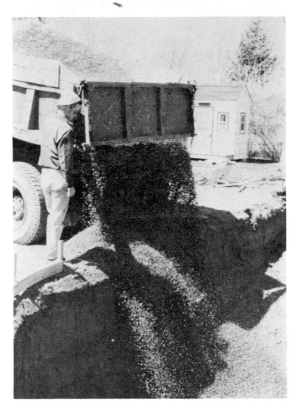

As soon as the hole is excavated, gravel is poured into it.

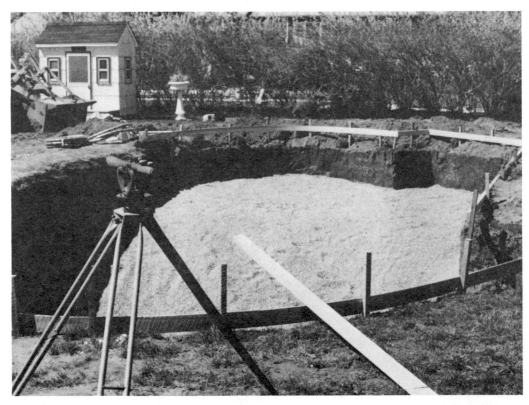

The gravel is spread over the bottom to form a stable support for the concrete that will form the pool sides and bottom.

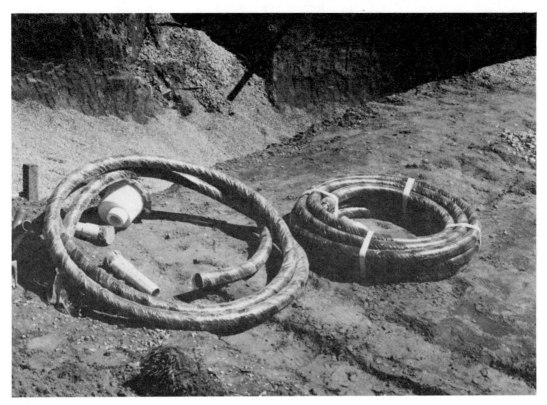

Once the gravel is down, the drain hoses can be laid in place. Pool drains used to be rigid pipe. Now they are 1½″ flexible PVC hose made specifically for pool, spa, and hot tub installations.

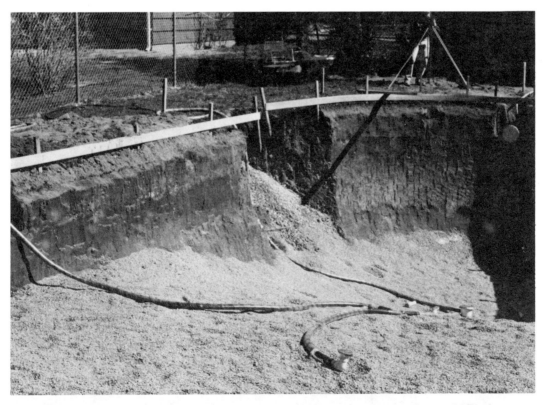

The hoses are attached to a main drain at the deepest point in the pool. Farther up the slope, toward the shallow end, are ports for the water returning to the pool. The hole in the side of the pool is where the septic tank was removed.

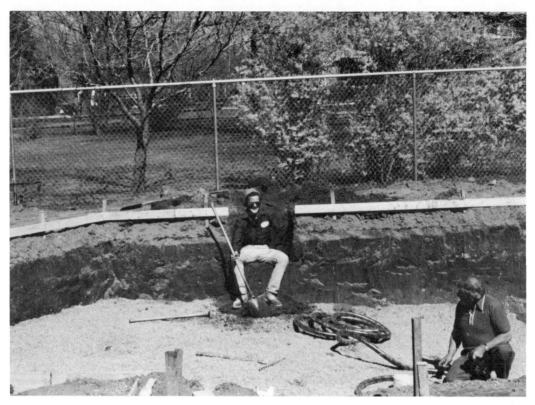

The hoses are laid to the edge of the pool and up to ground level via the recesses (where the workman is sitting) cut for the skimmers.

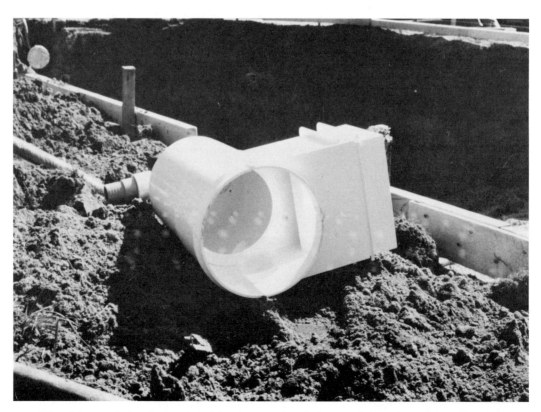

The skimmer is left beside its niche for the time being, to be set in place at the time the pool is given its cement shell.

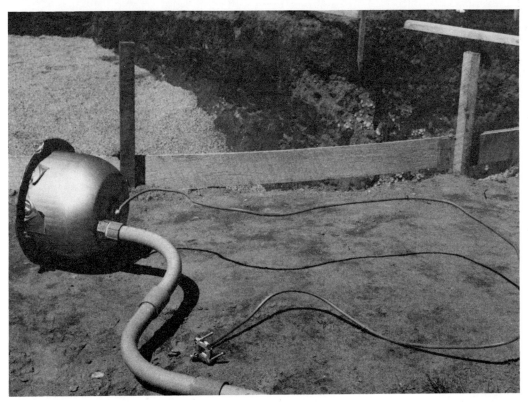

Another item installed now is the underwater light shell. An electrical cable runs through the curved pipe; the wire is a grounding wire.

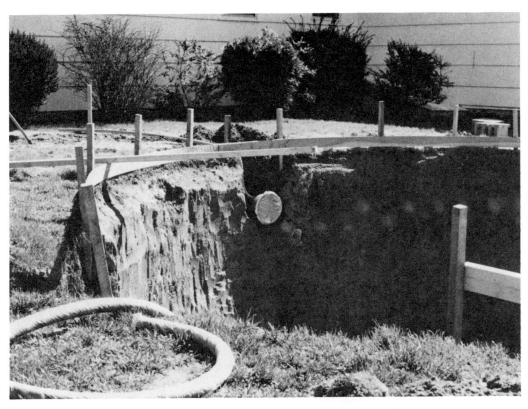

The lamp holder is positioned in its niche and covered with masking tape to prevent the concrete from entering it.

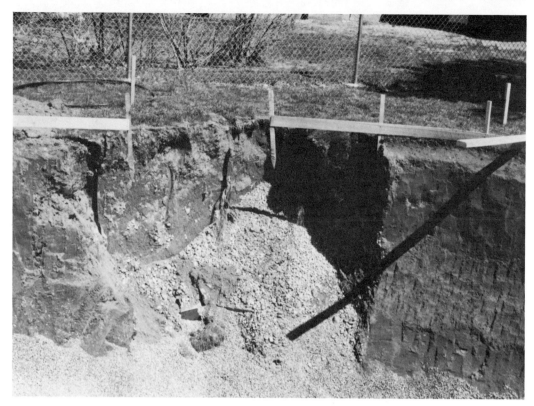

Before the Gunite crew can begin its work the pool must be shaped in front of the hole left by the septic tank. Unfortunately, the septic tank was at a point where the pool is supposed to curve.

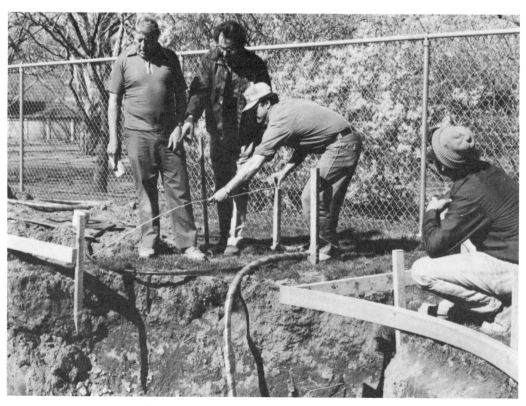

To establish the curve, careful measurements are taken . . .

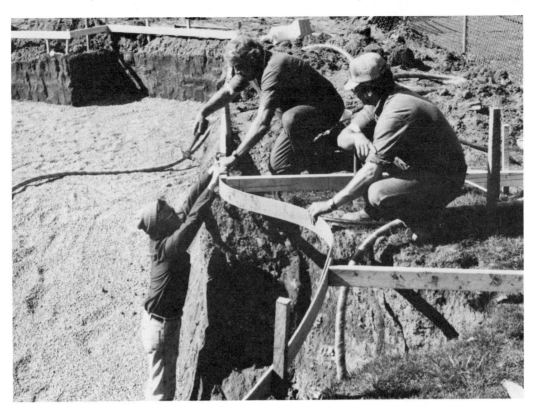

. . . and the framing is bent around the curve that the pool side will take.

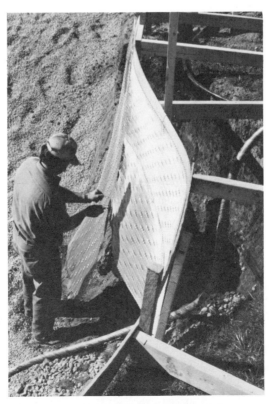

A wire mesh is then attached to the framing so that a minimum amount of Gunite will be blown into the hole and the pool will take its proper shape.

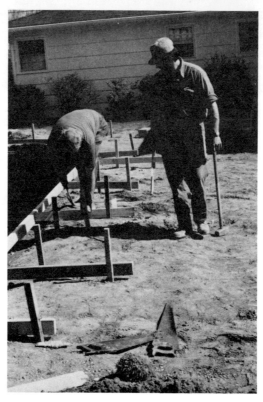

The framing around the edge of the pool must be reinforced at whatever points it is weak, because it will take a tremendous beating during the Gunite process.

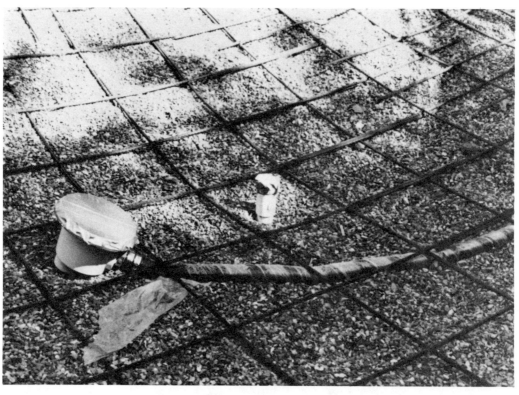

A mesh made of ⅜″ steel rods spaced every six inches is now laid across the bottom of the pool . . .

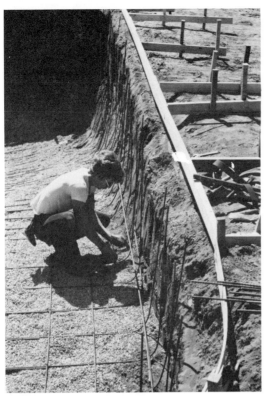

. . . and up the sides.

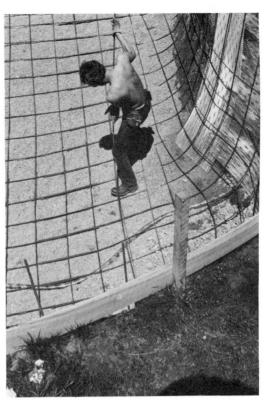

The rods are easily bent by leaning on them.

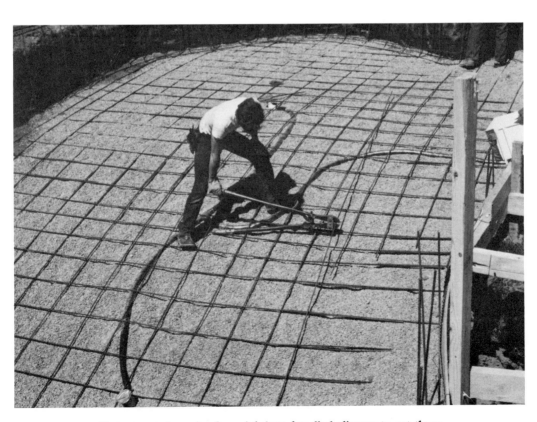

But you need a pair of special, long-handled clippers to cut them.

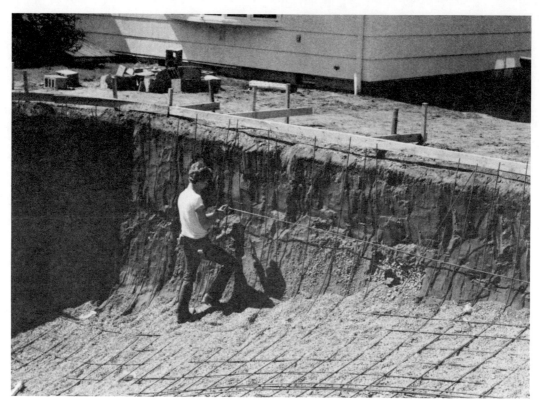

Every third or fourth rod that a given rod crosses is tied to it with baling wire.

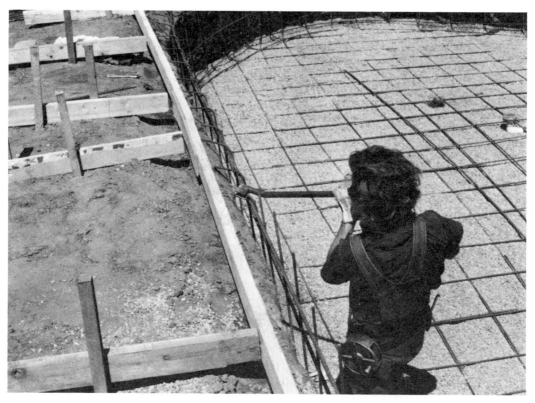

The tops of the side rods are wired to a ½″ steel rod and are then bent over it to form the top ledge of the pool.

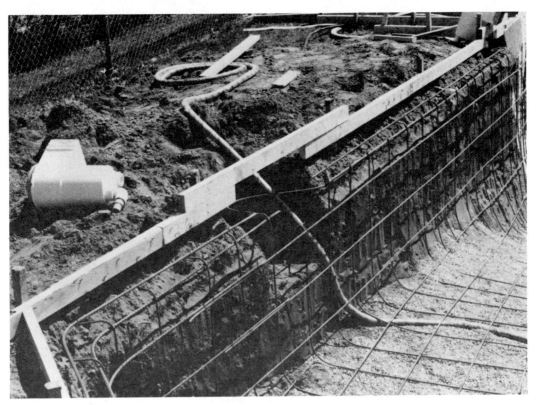

It takes two men less than four hours to place the rods for an average-sized pool. But if you have never done any rodding before, plan on at least two working days.

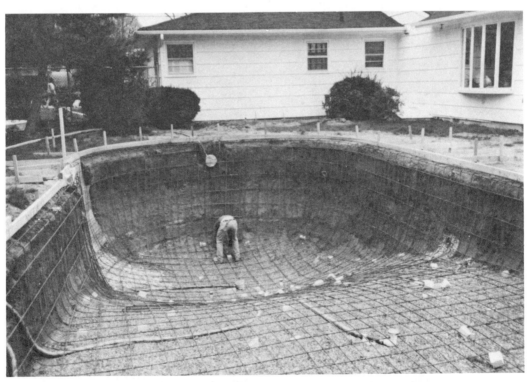

When the steel cage has been completed, it is suspended above the gravel by a series of concrete blocks, to allow the Gunite to flow underneath the metal. In other words, the cage will be in the middle of the Gunite shell, not around its outside.

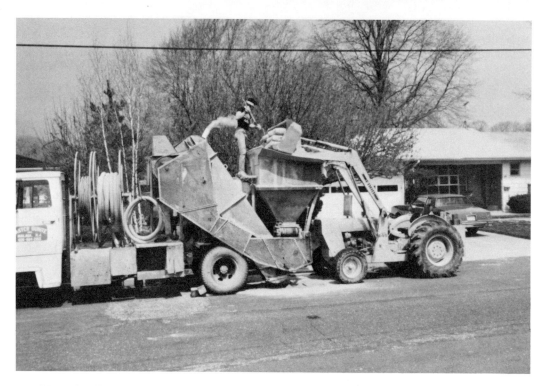

Now the big machinery arrives and the Gunite, which is a form of concrete, must be mixed to a consistency that can be blown through hoses (behind the cab of the truck) into the pool.

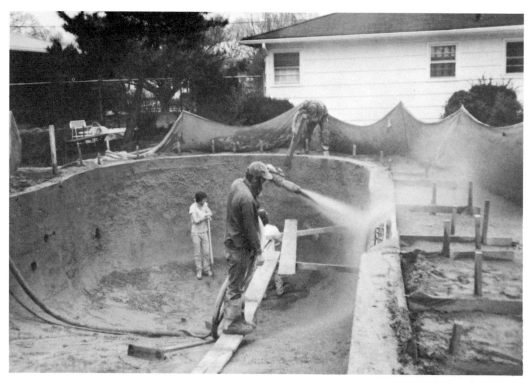

The Gunite process consumes the better part of a day. Once the concrete has been forced around the rods, its surface must be brushed even.

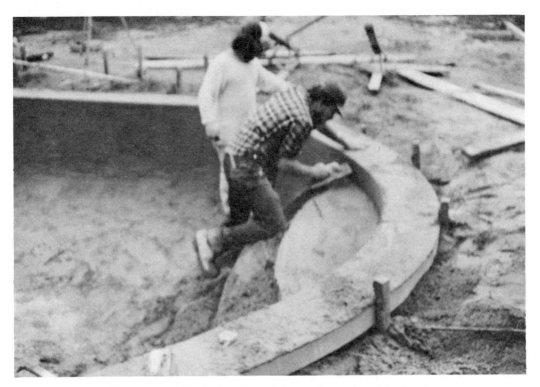

The steps at the shallow end of the pool are shaped by hand.

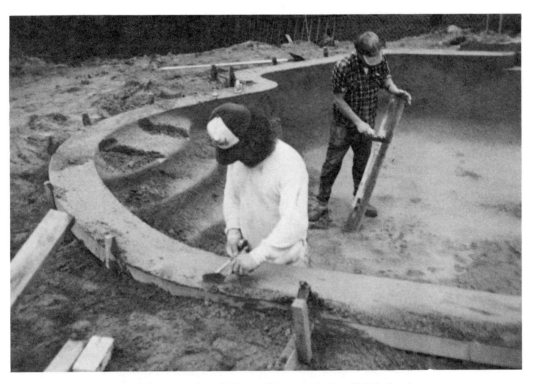

And the top edge of the pool is troweled until it is level.

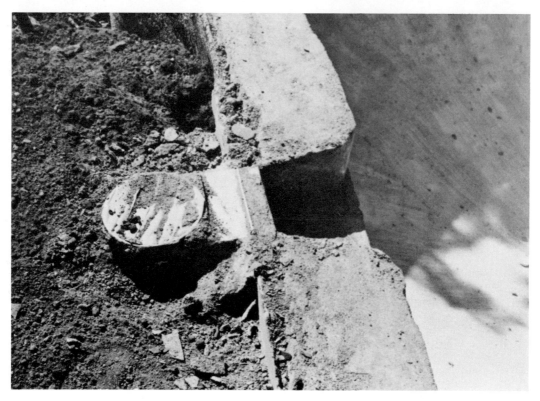

The skimmers have been set in place during the Gunite process and so have the step holes for the ladder, the underwater light . . .

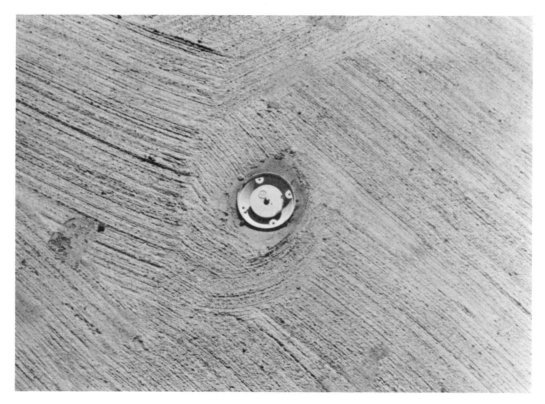

. . . and the drains. Note that the surface of the Gunite is left rough, so that the plaster that will go over it has a coarse surface to cling to.

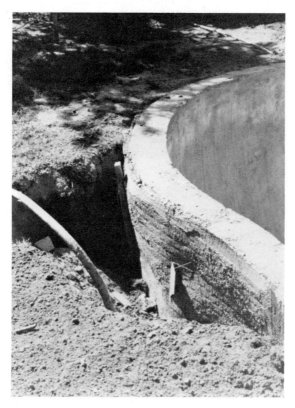

The curve of the pool across the front of the hole left by the septic tank now has a solid concrete face and can easily be backfilled with dirt.

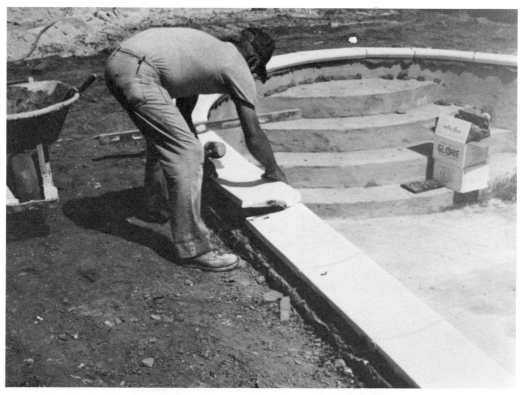

The Gunite must be allowed to set for about a week, and then curved edging blocks are cemented around the rim of the pool.

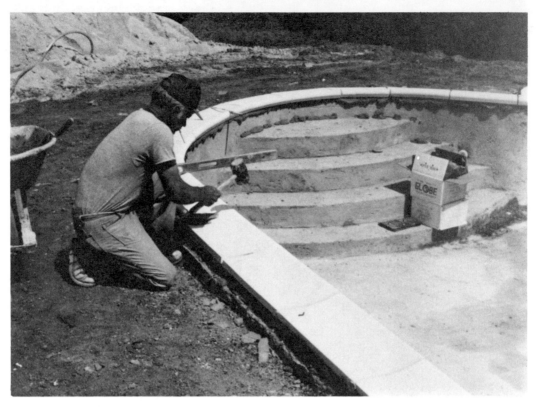

Each edging block must be tapped in place and leveled. Then the joints between blocks are filled with cement.

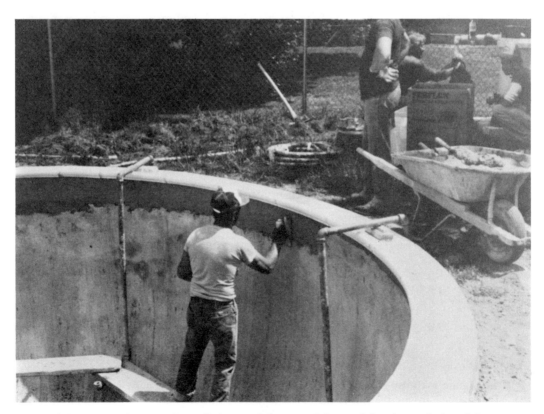

A base coat of cement is applied around the top of the pool, just beneath the edging.

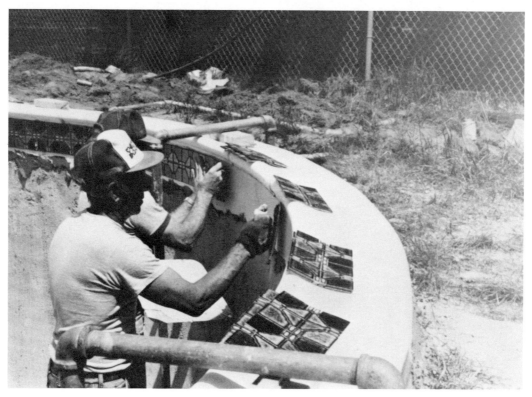

Next, a coat of fast-drying cement is spread over the base coat and the 6″ wide tile band is applied directly under the edging.

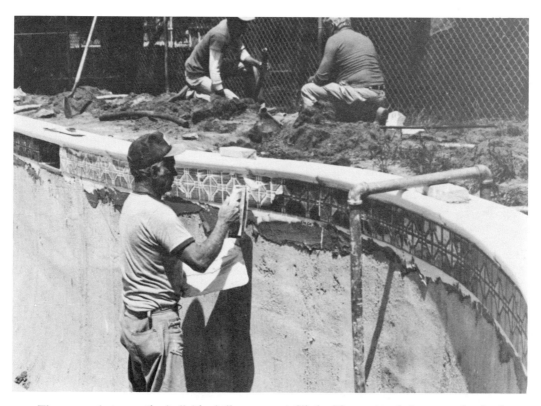

The spaces between the individual tiles are next filled with grout and the excess is wiped off the face of the tile.

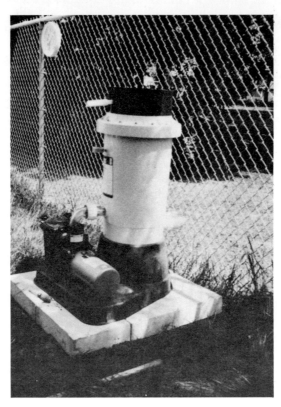

The filter, with its pump and motor, is installed on a concrete block plate at the same time the edging and tile are applied.

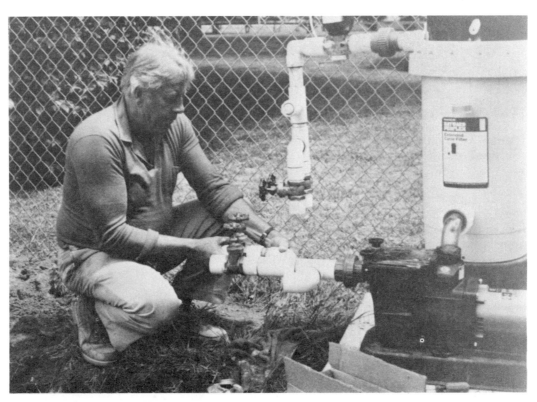

PVC pipes with shutoff valves for each incoming and outgoing line are connected to the filter and pump.

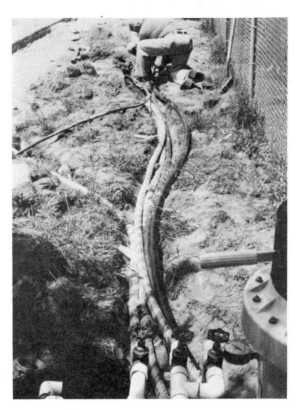

And the flexible PVC circulating pipes from the pool are connected at each valve. The pipes run from the main drain and the two skimmers to the pump, and water is returned to the pool through two return lines leading from the filter.

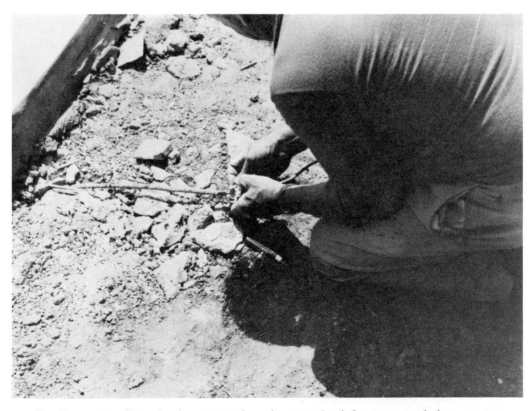

Finally, a grounding wire is connected to the central reinforcement rod that emerges from the pool at the shallow end.

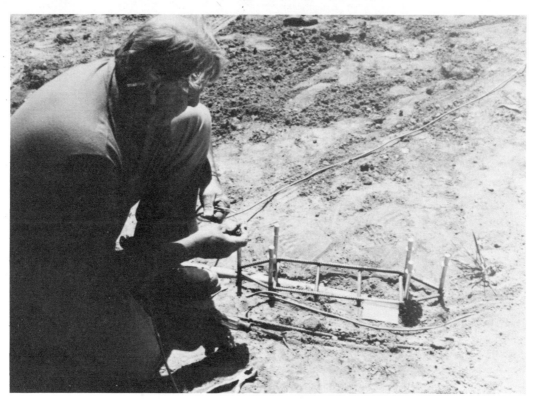

The grounding wire also connects to the pool ladder and the diving board, as well as the underwater light. Then it is attached to the other end of the same reinforcement rod as it emerges from the deep end of the pool. Thus, all of the metal attending the pool is grounded to the pool itself, providing a considerable margin of safety from electrical shock at all times.

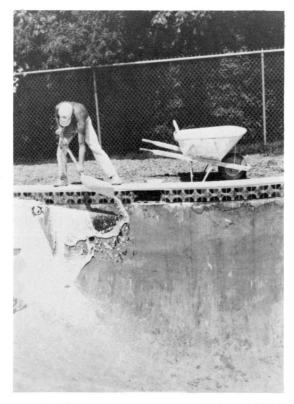

The plaster is composed of limestone, cement, and calcium, which dries quickly to a very hard surface. It is splashed against the sides of the pool.

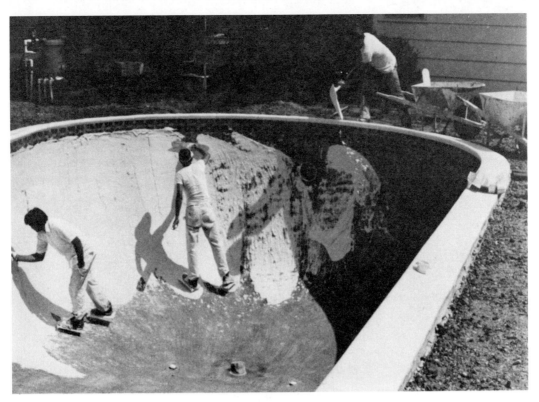

The plasterers work at a breakneck, nonstop pace, spreading the plaster on the concrete in two layers that produce a thickness of ⅜″.

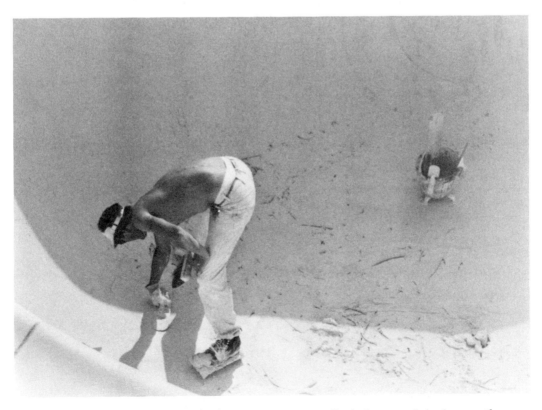

At first, while the plaster is still soft, the men wear spiked plates on their shoes as they smooth the plaster.

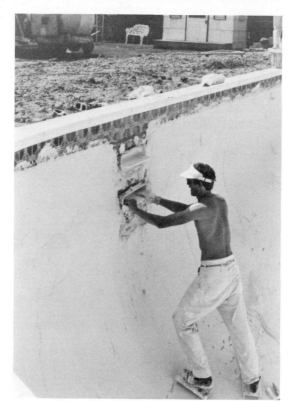

The vinyl steps for the ladder are filled with plaster and imbedded in their niches.

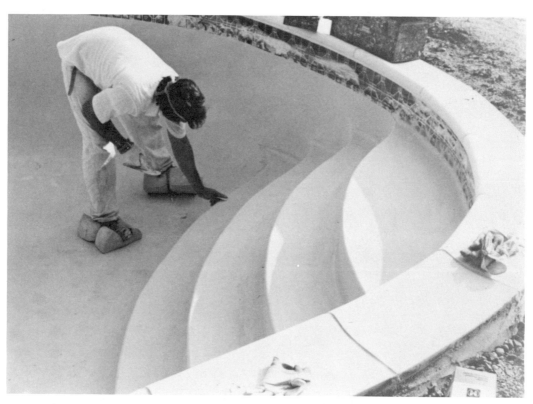

Within three hours the workers exchange their spikes for large sponges and move about the nearly hard surface troweling it into a smooth surface.

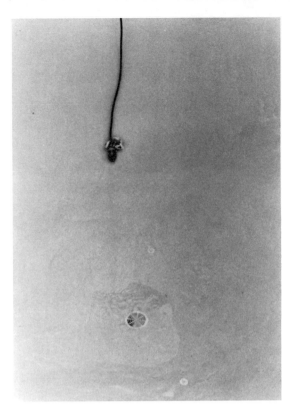

Water is pumped into the pool via a garden hose muzzled by a towel so that the splashing water will not mar the plaster surface.

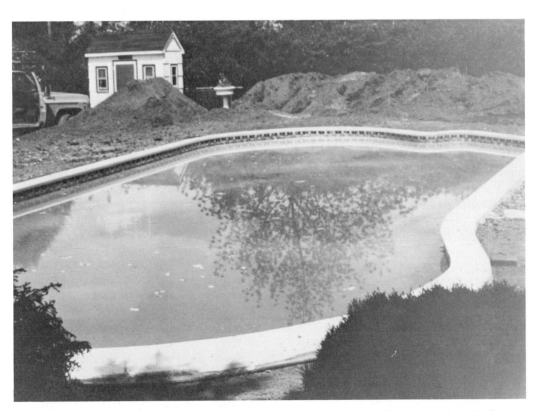

The plaster must be allowed to harden under water so that it will not develop checks or surface cracks. The diving board and ladder must be installed, and the water must be purified by chemicals and the filter system. But essentially, the Gunite swimming pool has been born.

CHAPTER FOUR

Pool Accessories

There are a dozen or so different accessories that you may want to consider adding to your pool as time goes by. You can spend about as much for all of them as the pool itself, so most people add accessories to their pools one or two at a time whenever their experience and budgets permit. As with most equipment, it is wisest to avoid buying products that cannot easily be serviced, or for which it is difficult to secure replacement parts. Also be wary of the cheaper products. Sometimes you can save a buck buying the least expensive version of a pool accessory and wind up spending more money in repairs or replacement than you would have spent with a better made, and therefore more expensive version.

There is no particular order in which pool accessories should be purchased; indeed, the order of priorities varies from pool owner to owner. Pool accessories would include:

A ladder and grab rails
A filter unit with a pump and motor
A water test kit
A pool brush or surface skimmer
A pool cover
A vacuum cleaner
An automatic surface skimmer

A diving board, stand, and/or slide
Underwater lights
Automatic cleaning system
Fencing
Automatic chemical feeder
Fences or windscreens
Chlorinator or Hypochlorinator

All of the above equipment can usually be purchased from your local pool supplier.

FILTERS

You cannot maintain the water in your swimming pool with any degree of clarity for more than about three days without pumping it through some kind of filter. Filters are designed to remove all of the fine particles of matter suspended in the water, because even if the water you use is absolutely clear when you put it in your pool, it will become clouded almost as soon as you begin using it.

If you do not have a filtration system supporting your pool, you will have to drain and scrub the pool every few days if you want the water to be at all clear, or you can extend the amount of time it takes the water to become turbid by add-

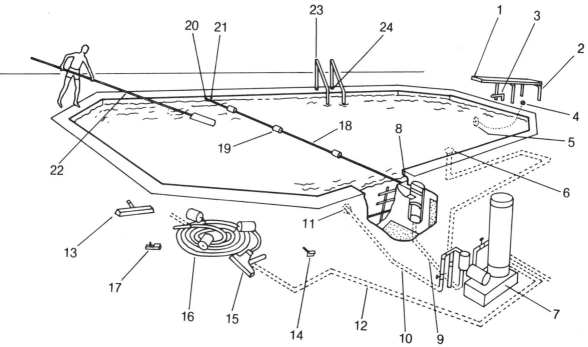

The accessories you can add to your pool include: 1. a diving board; 2. the diving board standards; 3. the pool fill spout; 4. the underwater light deck box; 5. an underwater light; 6. the main drain and suction section; 7. the filter; 8. an automatic skimmer; 9. the skimmer suction line; 10. the vacuum suction line; 11. the vacuum fitting; 12. the filter return line; 13. a pool brush; 14. a special algae brush; 15. the vacuum head; 16. the vacuum hose and floats; 17. a water test kit; 18. a pool life line; 19. the life line floats; 20. life line anchor hooks; 21. a rope hook (for the anchor hooks); 22. surface skimmer; 23. a wedge anchor and escutcheon; 24. a pool ladder.

ing chemicals to sterilize the water and break up parts of the suspended matter. But that is really only a stopgap method and considering the price of chemicals, it probably comes out costing more than installing and operating a filtering system.

There are three basic types of filters used in residential pools today. Sand filters represent the most popular form, followed by diatomaceous earth filters, and then cartridge filters. Which type you should use with your pool is ultimately up to you; you can find champions as well as detractors for all three types. But at least you can be reasonably certain that whatever type you ultimately purchase will do the job it is designed to do—keep your water bright and clear.

SAND FILTERS

Sand filters consist of a tank containing a foot or more of fine sand. Water from the pool is pumped into the tank and forced down through the sand, which traps the suspended impurities in the water before it is allowed to flow back into the pool via a return pipe. The pump and its controlling motor are mounted on the outside of the filter canister, along with a pressure gauge and a leaf strainer. When the sand in the filter becomes partially clogged (that is, saturated by debris), the water flow will be restricted and the unit's back pressure will rise above the normal 15 pounds per square inch (psi). The filter will then have to be back-flushed.

Back-flushing sand filters is a matter of rotating a directional valve so that water coming from the pool will be drawn through the sand in the opposite direction from the one that it usually travels. Then you turn on the pump and flush the debris out of the filter through a waste hose. Turn off the pump when the water leaving the filter turns clear; the filter is now cleaned and

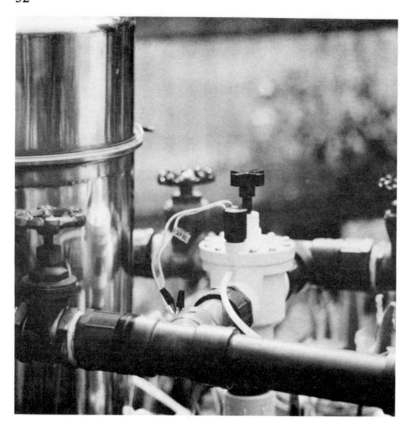

A filter system used with a small on-ground pool need not be very large.

you can resume the normal filtration process by turning the directional valve back to its original position and starting the pump again.

Sand filters are regulated to permit a flow of between 3 and 5 gallons of water per minute per square foot of filter area. The backwash pipe must be connected to a hose or pipe leading to a sewer line or some other means of releasing the several hundred gallons of water needed to clean out the filter. The sand used in sand filters can be any of several types specified by the manufacturer of the unit, although it is usually some form of silica. The great advantage to sand filters is their longevity and ease of maintenance; they have been known to last for a score of years before needing repair or replacement.

DIATOMITE EARTH FILTERS

This type of filter uses a fabric element (usually a synthetic such as Orlon) as a diaphragm that the water must pass through. Diatomaceous earth, which is a powdery substance consisting of microscopic siliceous skeletons, is placed in the filter tank to form a porous coating on the ele-

ment and acts as a filter for the water, entrapping a large portion of the suspended substances in the water. There are two general categories of diatomite filters, pressure and vacuum types.

PRESSURE DIATOMITE FILTERS

The pressure versions of diatomite filters employ a bag inside a pressure tank. The pool water is pumped into the top of the filter, passes through the bag, which is coated with diatomaceous earth, that filters it before it re-enters the pool. This type of filter must be opened from time to time to launder or replace the bag.

PRESSURE LEAF FILTERS

These employ flat leaves or several spirally wound elements to provide the most possible filter area in the least possible space. The elements are separated by a noncorrosive mesh and are coated with diatomaceous earth. The elements can usually be cleaned with a hose spray once the lid of the filter is removed. This type of filter is popular with smaller on-ground or portable pools and is considered to have the longest filter cycle of any of the filters.

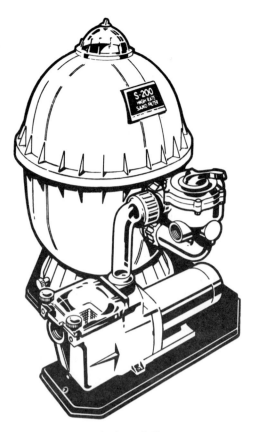

A typical sand filter.

Vacuum diatomaceous earth filters function pretty much the same as pressure leaf filters. However, the filter pump is connected to the return side of the filter so that instead of pushing water through the unit, the pump sucks it through. The sucking action allows the filter to be used in conjunction with a skimmer, with the advantage that you have one machine doing the work of two, drawing the pool water from the surface, sucking it through the diatomaceous leaves, and returning it to the pool. There is normally an adjustment on the filter that allows you to draw water from the main pool drain or the vacuum outlet whenever you are brushing or vacuum cleaning the pool.

CARTRIDGE FILTERS

Cartridge filters consist of a tank containing one or several replaceable cartridges that may be made of porous stone, cotton, stainless steel, and/or plastic. Water from the pool is forced into the tank and through the cartridge elements, then out of the tank again. Whenever the cartridges become clogged with sediment, they are simply discarded and replaced, a chore that takes but a few minutes to complete.

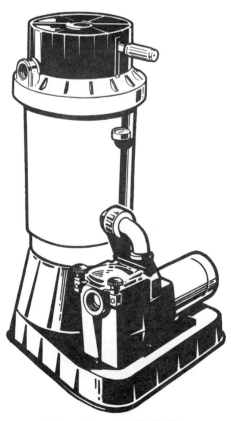

A diatomite earth (DE) filter.

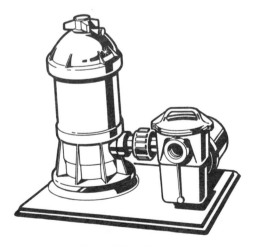

A cartridge filter.

SELECTING A FILTER

Whatever filter you choose, the most important factor to consider is the volume of water it must handle. While the filter should be large enough to handle the capacity of your pool, it is more energy efficient to have a filter that is too large than one that is not capable of filtering the entire contents of the pool every fourteen to eighteen hours. However, a considerably shorter filter cycle is not only inadequate, but will add to your installation and maintenance costs, so you really want to come as close as possible to matching the capacity of the filter with the volume of water to be filtered.

FIGURING POOL VOLUMES

Before you begin shopping for a pool filter, know how much the volume of water is in your pool. To compute that volume in terms of gallons of water, use this formula:

length $\times$ width $\times$ average depth $\times$ 7.47 $=$ gallons

The length and width of the pool are easily measured. Finding the average depth is a little more complicated. In general, a pool designed for diving will average 6 feet in depth, but if you want to be more exact, use the average depth in each depth section and figure the cubic area for each portion, then add them all together. The 7.47 figure is the number of gallons that can be contained in an area that is $1' \times 1' \times 1'$. Thus, a $20' \times 40'$ pool with an average depth of $6'$ is computed in this manner:

$40'$ (length) $\times$ $20'$ (width) $\times$ average depth ($6'$) $=$ 4800 cubic feet
4800 cubic feet $\times$ 7.47 (gallons per cubic feet) $=$ 35,856 gallons

In order to filter that much water in a fourteen- to eighteen-hour period, the filter you purchase will have to be able to pass between 33 and 43 gallons per minute (gpm) through its tank, and its filter capacity should be such that the filter does not need to be cleaned more often than every four days during normal operating conditions.

FILTER SYSTEM COMPONENTS

Filters come in tanks. Attached to the outside of the tank are several components, all of which are important to the operation of the filter. There should be influent and affluent pressure gauges which register the pressure differential inside the tank and tell you when you have to clean the filter. The normal pressure level is around 15 psi and is stamped on the manufacturer's data plate, but this 15 psi will rise as the filter becomes clogged with dirt, giving you an indication of when the filter must be cleaned or replaced.

The system will also have an air release valve at its highest point to protect it from too much pressure, and there should be a visual means of determining when the filter is producing clean water. This visual means is normally in the form of a glass (or plastic) container that you can look into and watch the water as it passes from the filter back to the pool.

The heart of any filter is, of course, its pump and motor, and as a rule these are sold as part of the filter package. The pump-motor must have enough capacity to provide the proper flow of water through the filter and, depending on the size of your pool and the rated flow through the filter, it can be anything from a ¼ to 3 hp single phase 60Hz 110/220 volt unit. Most filter pumps are centrifugal types and self-priming. As a self-primer, the pump does not require a pump pit and may be installed anywhere near the filter. Moreover, it will automatically expel any air that gets into the lines, preventing air-lock in the recirculating pipes.

Modern electric motors and the centrifugal pumps they operate require little or no maintenance. Some types may need an occasional oiling, although most are sealed units that do not even need that. You will probably be running the motor between four and eight hours a day during the swimming season, but you can expect something around seven years of use before the motor and/or pump need replacement, and conceivably even at that point the units may only need some replacement parts or merely basic servicing. You do have to be careful that the wiring from the motor is properly made and that the circuit that feeds the motor is protected by a Ground Fault Circuit Interrupter (GFCI).

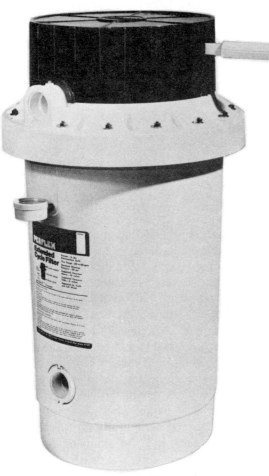

A filter tank.

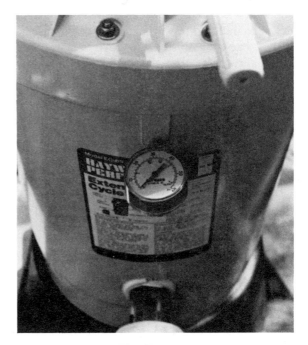

The filter gauges.

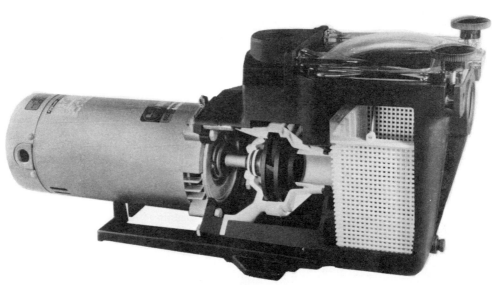

The filter pump and its motor.

WHAT A FILTER SYSTEM CAN DO FOR YOU

The proper-sized filter when correctly operated and maintained will provide you with clear water and is considered a "must" accessory for any swimming pool since it removes all of the solids suspended in the water. It removes the solids but not perspiration, urine, saliva, suntan lotion, cosmetics, bacteria, viruses, and, in particular, algae. All of these can accumulate and cause the water to become murky; to keep all of them under control you have to use oxidizing agents and algae inhibitors, which are injected into the water every few days or so.

WATER TEST KITS

Even if you do not have a filter system attached to your pool, it is practically mandatory to possess—and use—a water test kit. The kit can be any of several brands found on the market, and the one you select should be easy to read accurately. It should also be capable of telling you when your water requires more chlorine and whether or not the water possesses the proper balance of acid and alkali. The kits are not

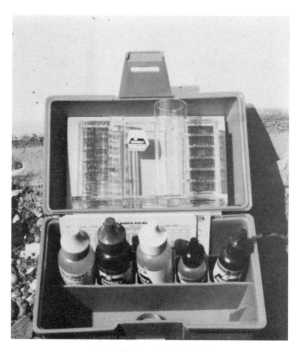

A typical water test kit.

difficult to use and can prevent your pool water from becoming chemically unsafe. A full discussion of test kits and how to use them with swimming pools will be found in Chapter Eight.

SKIMMERS

There are two types of skimmers used with swimming pools; it is recommended that at least one skimming device be installed for every 800 square feet of water surface. One type is built into the pool during its construction, while the other is a separate unit that works off a vacuum line. In both cases, the skimmer functions as a catch-all for relatively large debris such as dust, skin particles, leaves, and hair that settle on the surface of the water. All of these tiny particles will eventually settle on the bottom of the pool, but the skimmer is designed to suck them into the filter before they can fall beneath the surface of the water. Built-in skimmers have a basket inside them which traps any really large debris as the surface water is drawn through it on its way to the filter. The basket obviously must be removed and cleaned periodically, just as the filter must be cleaned; and the skimmer should be turned off during the filter backwash operation so that the filter does not flush itself back into the pool.

The vacuum type of skimmer operates in the same manner as its built-in brethren, except it is plugged into the pool vacuum line.

CLEANING EQUIPMENT

While a long-handled pool brush is invaluable for cleaning algae from the sides and floor of a pool, it will usually cause the tiniest, lightest dirt particles to be stirred up in the water. The majority of the dirt scraped off the pool walls can be pushed toward the main drain where it will be sucked into the filter to be disposed of later. But you still have those minute particles floating around in the water, so a more efficient method of cleaning your pool is with a vacuum cleaner.

VACUUM CLEANERS

Pools having a recirculating filter normally are equipped with a vacuum outlet into the pool during its construction. The outlet is connected directly to the filter system via a pipe and can

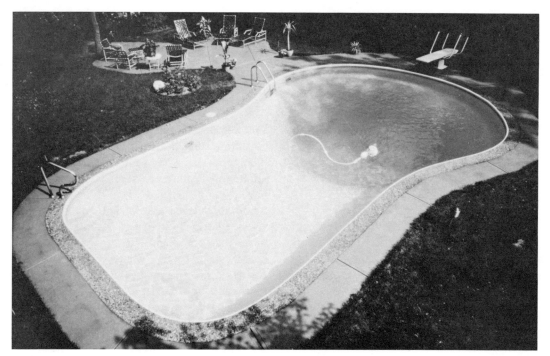

A vacuum-type skimmer is plugged into the vacuum line and simply floats around on the surface of the pool.

therefore use the filter pump and pump strainer attached to the filter. Normally, when the vacuum is in use, all leaves and large debris taken from the water are trapped in the pump strainer and all of the finer particles in the water are left in the filter as water is vacuumed from the pool.

The vacuum itself consists of a cleaning head on wheels that contains a brush. The head is attached to a long aluminum handle, allowing you to clean the pool floor from the surrounding pool deck. There is also a suction hose connected to the cleaning head at one end, and the vacuum outlet at the other, which draws whatever water and debris the head moves over into the filter system.

There is only one point of caution to remember when using a pool vacuum. The hose must be completely filled with water before the unit is turned on so that no air can get into the pump and cause the pump to malfunction.

There is a variety of vacuums available at pool dealers and supply outlets. One version uses a hydraulic water-pressure principle instead of a pump and can be used on pools that do not have a vacuum outlet. The jet-type cleaners consist of

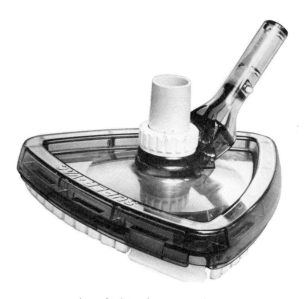

A typical pool vacuum cleaner.

a cleaning head attached to a hose leading to a water supply faucet. Water from the faucet enters the nozzle under a normal 45 to 60 psi, causing a pressure in the cleaner that creates a vacuum which sucks pool water up to the filter bag and back into the pool again, once it has been cleaned. While this type of vacuum cleaner is not as efficient as the pump-operated types, it will do an adequate job of cleaning your pool, and it is generally a less expensive piece of equipment.

STEPS AND LADDERS

Steps or ladders are provided at the shallow end of any pool if the vertical distance from the bottom of the pool to the deck or the top of the pool wall is more than 2′ and/or if the deep end exceeds 5′ in depth. If the pool is more than 40′ long, there should be a second set of steps or a ladder to serve the deep end of the unit. Any pool that is more than 30′ wide at the deep end should also have steps or ladders installed at each side.

STEPS

When you are building a pool and decide to incorporate steps in its ends or sides, you can make them any size you want, so long as they meet minimum requirements. All step treads must have an unobstructed width of at least 10″ and a minimum surface area of 240 square inches. The risers, that is the height, of each step must be no more than 12″ high and all of the steps have to be the same height, whatever it may be. If the treads do not end against a side wall of the pool, there must be a handrail or grab rail.

If the steps are inserted in the pool wall, the step holes should be sloped to drain into the pool

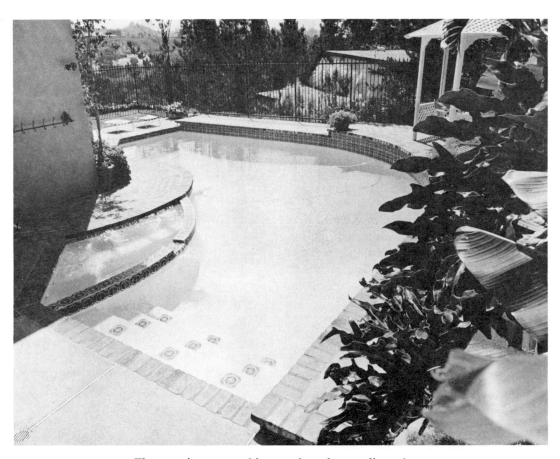

The steps incorporated in a pool can be any dimension.

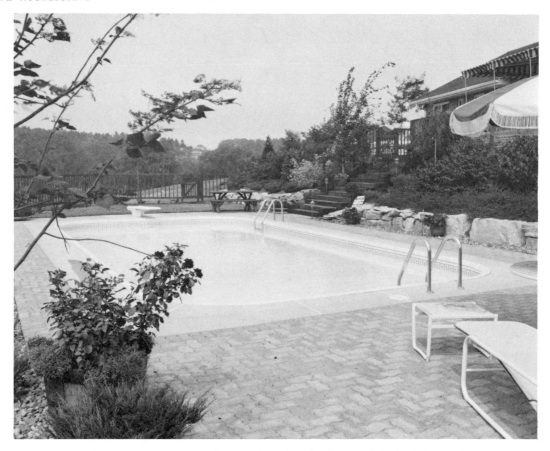

Pool ladders must be solidly anchored to the sides and deck of the pool.

so that dirt cannot accumulate in them. Step holes should be at least 5″ deep and 12″ wide and be provided with a grab rail at both sides of the treads.

LADDERS

Pool ladders that are affixed to the sides of a pool are made of corrosion resistant material and have nonslip treads. All ladders are designed with handrails which must be securely installed with a clearance of no more than 6″ and no less than 3″ from the wall where they are attached.

Portable pool ladders used for egress to above-ground pools must extend above the top of the pool wall or the surrounding pool deck by at least 20″. They must have slip resistant treads and be provided with side rails. They are all constructed to be as stable as possible, but that stability can only be the partial responsibility of the manufacturer. The ladder can be built like a rock

and still be unsafe if it is not located on a solid base that guarantees it will stay absolutely plumb. There are also some safety rules that should be imposed on anyone using a portable ladder:

1. Always face the ladder when climbing up or down it.

2. Only one person should ever be on the ladder at any one time.

3. No one should jump or dive from the ladder.

4. Portable ladders should be removed from the pool when they are not in use.

DIVING EQUIPMENT

Diving equipment includes high and low boards, diving stands, and slides. It goes without saying that whatever the diving equipment, it must be substantially constructed to support the unusual

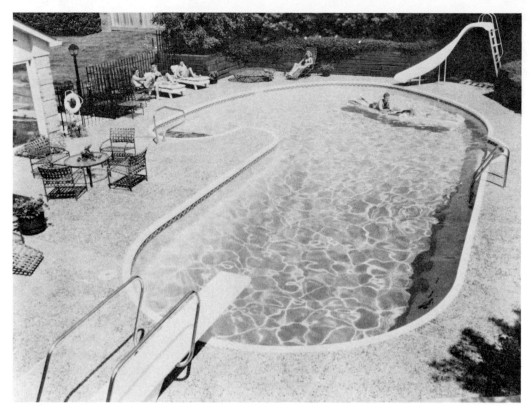

Diving equipment includes boards and slides and stands.

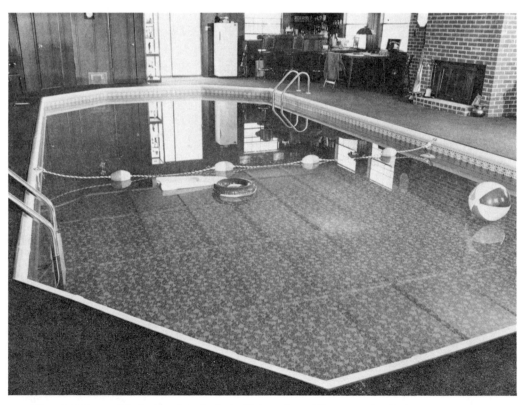

If an indoor pool is designed to include diving, the ceiling must be high enough so that divers do not hurt themselves.

weights and stresses. It must also be permanently installed and, if the pool is roofed, there must be ample head room above it. The length of the board and its height above the water depends on the type of pool you own:

Pool Type	Head Room	Max. Diving Board Length	Max. Jump Board Length	Max. Board Height Over Water
I	NO DIVING EQUIPMENT PERMITTED			
II	12'	8'	6'	½ meter (20")
III	12'	10'	8'	⅔ meter (26")
IV	13'	12'	8'	¾ meter (30")
V	14'	12'	8'	1 meter (40")

Slides must also be permanently anchored to the pool deck and positioned at the edge of the water so that all water flowing off the slide will enter the pool. The slide must be positioned so that the center line of the slide does not intersect with the center line of the nearest diving board for at least 7' in front of the board. All sides must be positioned so that no slide user can touch the edge of the pool, a diving board, or anything else with his or her arms extended.

SAFEGUARDS

The realm of pool safety takes you into such accessories as a safety line, a life line and life ring, a pool cover, and handholds.

HANDHOLDS

A suitable handhold is required around the perimeter of any area where the depth exceeds 3'6". Such handholds should be no farther apart than every 4', but they can be any one or combination of several things. You can have a coping, ledge, or a deck that is no more than 1' above the water line. You can have ladders, steps, or seat ledges. A seat, when it is provided, cannot be more than 20" below the water line. Alternatively, you can have a rope or railing placed not more than 12" above the water line and fastened to a wall of the pool. Given the tendency to pro-

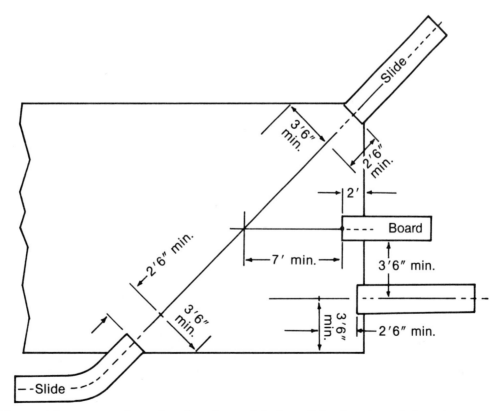

Slides must be permanently anchored to the pool deck as diving boards, and the units must be kept well away from each other, to prevent injury to divers.

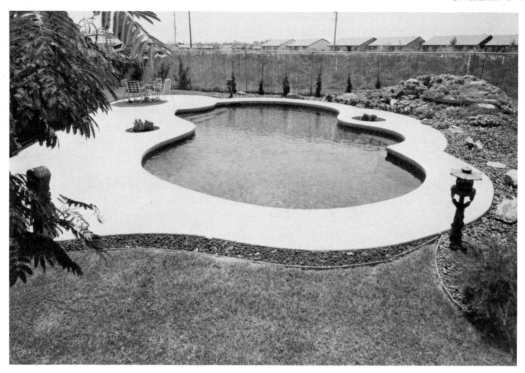

The deck around most in-ground pools becomes an automatic handhold.

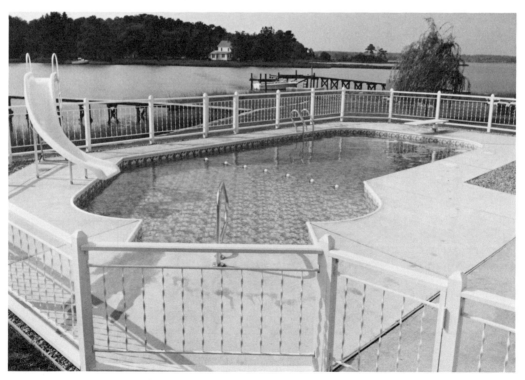

A safety line is usually anchored across the pool at the point where its depth increases. The line must be kept above the water surface by floats.

vide a decking around most pools, as well as a coping over the top of the walls, a "suitable handhold" is almost automatically a part of every in-ground pool.

SAFETY LINES

Pool safety lines must be permanently attached across the width of the pool and be supported by buoys, since they must be installed at, or slightly above, the water line. The line is normally installed at the end of the wading area to separate it from deep water to alert nonswimmers as to where their boundaries of safety end. The line itself is usually a synthetic fiber rope supported by Styrofoam buoys. Since both materials lend themselves to bright colors and resist water damage, they will remain strong for several seasons.

SAFETY ACCESSORIES

One recommended safety accessory is a good-quality life ring that has an approved Coast Guard rating (Type IV personnel flotation device). This is technically known as a life ring buoy and may be made of cork, balsa wood, or a unicellular plastic foam. Life rings come in 18½", 20", 24", and 36" diameter sizes and are marked as acceptable throwable devices.

The rings have an obvious safety value; a shepherd's crook with its 12′ handle is an equally handy safety device, but it is also useful for fishing objects out of the pool and for teaching beginners good swimming techniques. There are no laws stating that you have to have one around, but it is a useful tool to own.

POOL COVERS

A pool cover may sound at first as though it should be on the bottom of your equipment list, but it has some value in ways that are not always obvious. To begin with, the covers are made of a light but very strong plastic that is easily rolled out over the water by one person. By putting it over the water whenever the pool is not in use, you will prevent dust and leaves from falling in the water, with the result that your maintenance work is simplified. Less obvious, it prevents the water from evaporating as quickly as it might otherwise, which saves water, a natural resource that in many parts of the country is often in short supply. In fact, by using a pool cover, you can save between 50 and 75 percent of the energy needed to heat your pool. Finally, the cover offers a safety factor in that it can support a 200-pound person, should he (or she) fall in the pool when the cover is in place over the water.

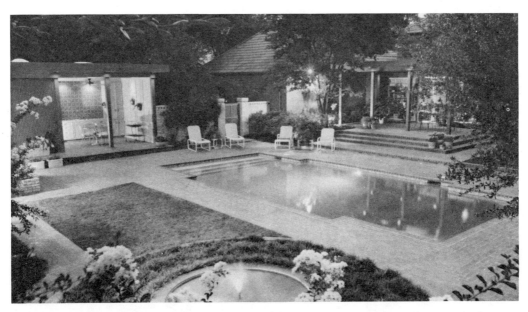

Even though a pool is well lit at night, it must still have underwater lights so that swimmers can see when they are beneath the surface.

Pool covers are so inexpensive they will pay for themselves in a single season.

UNDERWATER LIGHTS

Underwater lighting has both a beautifying as well as a safety purpose. If you incorporate underwater lighting, it must be allowed for during the planning stages since the lights are placed in recesses in the pool walls, typically 3′ below the water line at the deep end of the pool. They may be removed and their bulbs changed without any danger from electrical hazard and are considerably safer than the old method of sealing a lamp behind glass fixed in the side of the pool.

The value of being able to light the water under its surface does not become apparent until you decide to have an evening swimming party. At that point, no matter how well the surface of the water is illuminated, swimmers will be unable to see obstacles (or other people) under water, reducing the margin of safety when they are swimming or diving. Prevent one injury, and the cost of including underwater lighting with your pool will have paid for itself.

CHAPTER FIVE

Heating a Swimming Pool

About half of the residential pools in America are equipped with heaters. The majority of these heated installations are in the northern climates, and while some of them are for the purpose of making the pool available throughout the winter, most are used merely to extend the swimming season by a month or two in the spring and again in the fall. There are countless days in the months of March, April, and May, and again in October and November, when it would be pleasant to take a dip in your pool—if the water were warm enough. If your pool does not have a heater, the days may be balmy enough, but the cold nights in between keep the swimming water too chilly for comfort.

The basic principle for heating a swimming pool remains the same whether you employ a direct heater or use a solar pool heating system. But heaters are expensive to install and to operate because they must consume a costly energy such as natural gas, fuel oil, or electricity.

If you think you might want a pool heater someday, plan for it (and make the space to house it) while you are building your pool. It is cheaper to install a heater as you build the pool, but if that represents too much of an added expense, at least make allowances for it during the pool construction. The heater needs to have inlet lines that are separate from the pipes going to and from the filter, and as a rule these pipe lines are buried underground. If you have to go to the expense of digging trenches to the pool and messing up your decking and landscaping at some future date, you may find yourself in a more complicated (and costly) situation than you want to deal with.

In general, gas- or oil-fired heaters are considered more efficient than electrical units; solar heating systems are practically free of operational costs, but they cost considerably more to install. And believe it or not, when it comes to pool heaters, "bigger is better." A pool needs the same amount of heat to raise the temperature of its water whether you deliver that heat quickly or over a long period of time. The drawback in taking a long time to heat your pool with a small heater is that you will have considerable heat loss during the warm-up period. In other words, a heater that is too small for the volume of water it must heat will have to work longer, and therefore will use more fuel. Furthermore, the water rapidly dissipates whatever heat it is given, so a

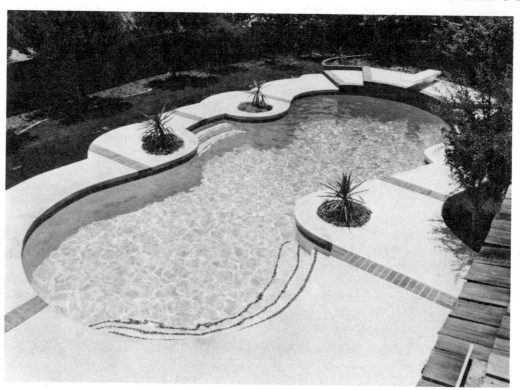

If your pool is equipped with a good heater, you can extend your swimming season by several months during the spring and fall.

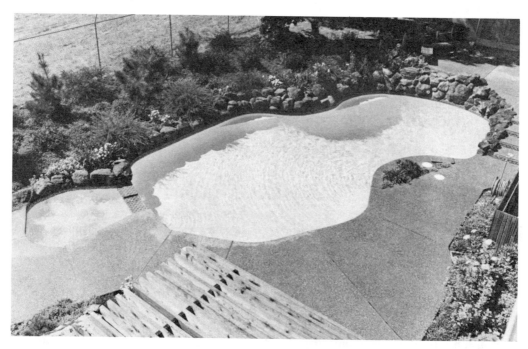

If your pool is connected to a spa, you will need two heaters, one for the pool and the other for the spa.

small heater has to keep plugging away for hours trying to get the temperature of the water up a few degrees. The professional recommendation for heaters is to install a unit that is big enough to get the pool temperature up to a comfortable level quickly. At that point, the heater closes down and stops using fuel for a while until the pool cools a few degrees. Another advantage of using a larger heater is that you can incorporate an on/off switch to heat the water quickly for special occasions such as a weekend or a party and use less energy than would be required to keep a constant temperature all of the time.

It has been established by the medical profession that the most beneficial temperature for healthful and recreational swimming is 78° F. Anything more than that and you are wasting energy and providing excessive heat, just as if you were overheating a room. Bear in mind that for every degree you raise your pool water above 78° F., you will increase your energy needs by 10 percent.

HEATING CONSERVATION

The National Swimming Pool Institute offers these suggestions for maintaining heated pools:

1. Extend your swimming season by a reasonable time. For example, if you heat your pool for three months instead of five, you can reduce your energy needs by 33 percent.

2. Set the heater thermostat control to 78° F. and don't let anyone tamper with it.

3. If you go away on vacation, or you are shutting the pool down for the winter, turn the heat completely off. This means shutting off the pilot light, if there is one.

4. Shelter your pool from prevailing breezes. You can do this with fences, windscreens, landscaping, anything that will reduce evaporation and heat loss.

5. Follow a regular program of preventive maintenance for the heater. There should be an annual inspection and the heat exchanger should be delimed whenever necessary.

DIRECT HEATERS

Natural gas, oil, and electricity are all used to operate standard pool heaters; and among the most common heaters used are the horizontal-

tube heater, the coil type, and the vertical-flue type. With the horizontal-tube type, water passes through a series of horizontal tubes positioned over an open-flame burner. The coil-type heaters have a coiled tube that carries the water through the heater over an open flame. The vertical-flue type has a series of vertical tubes positioned over open flames. Essentially, all three types have an open fire at the base which licks away at the pipes above it, heating whatever water is passing

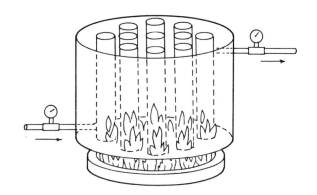

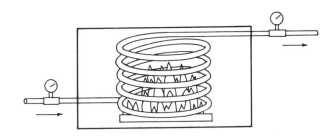

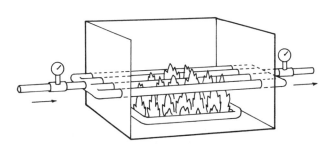

The three most common heaters are the vertical-flue type (top), the coil type (middle), and the horizontal-tube type.

through them. Typically, the water is brought to the heater as soon as it leaves the pool filter and is returned to the pool as soon as it has been heated.

No matter what type of heater you are using, it should be equipped with both an aquastat and a thermometer. The aquastat controls the heat in the heater relative to the temperature you want the water in the pool to be. The thermometer tells you how hot the heated water is. Most units also have a "high-limit" control that automatically shuts down the heater whenever it begins operating in too hot a range, and a pressure control regulator that will immediately turn off the heater if there is no water pressure in the pipes, coils, or flues.

Some heaters have a thermometer at both the input and output lines of the boiler so that you can always be sure the heated water is the proper temperature. The desired differential between the cool water entering the heater and the heated water leaving it is 30° F. Thus, the heater should be delivering heated water back to the pool that is 30° above the temperature you want the pool water to maintain. If the desired temperature is the recommended 78° F., the water leaving the heater will be 108° F. The reason for a 30° differential is that the ratio will produce a minimum amount of condensation and boiler scale, so it is a critical temperature to maintain at all times.

Heaters should be installed in a well-ventilated room that provides air circulation around the unit, so there will be a sufficient supply of oxygen to allow it to operate at peak efficiency. To generate this air circulation, there should be at least two vents that are each 2½ square feet.

Remember that the heater is in operation

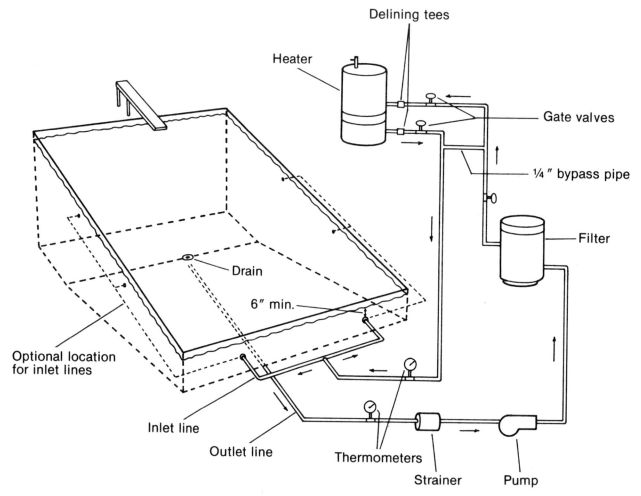

Anatomy of a pool supported by a heater and filter.

whenever the filter is running. It is possible to close a cut-off valve in the pipe leading from the filter to divert the filtered water back into the pool without heating it, but any time you need the heater the water first goes through the filter. As a result, when you are initially warming up the pool it may be necessary to run the filter for longer periods of time than is normal. You might even have to run both units around the clock if the water is really cold.

HEATER SIZES

The rule that is applied when deciding the size of a heater is this: Below 1,000' above sea level, allow 8 BTU's per gallon of water to be heated. A BTU is a British Thermal Unit and is defined as the amount of heat needed to raise the temperature of 1 pound of water 1° per hour. As an example, if you have a 20' × 40' pool containing 35,856 gallons of water, and you need a heater that can deliver 8 BTU's per hour, multiply 8 BTU's by 35,856 gallons. Now you know that the heater must have a capacity rating of 286,848 BTU's to raise the temperature of the pool approximately 1° per hour. This is, however, a rule of thumb. In order to determine accurately the size and type of unit you will need, also consider the altitude above sea level at which your pool is situated, the amount of use the heater will get, the size and type of filter you are installing, even the micro-climate of the pool itself and the type of water you are using. The balancing of all these factors is relatively complicated and is best done by an expert such as your local pool dealer or contractor.

MAINTAINING HEATERS

A direct pool heater is not really very different in its operation and maintenance from a standard hot water heater, and it should be accorded the same treatment as your hot water heater. The pool heater should be inspected and serviced annually as a matter of course. In areas where the water is unusually hard, you may find the boiler has to be cleaned several times a year to prevent the buildup of calcium scale. The calcium in your water supply, if it is allowed to accumulate, will drastically reduce the efficiency of any heater, and keeping the boiler clean is the only effective way of preventing trouble. It is possible,

in extreme situations, to inject a sequestering agent such as sodium hexametaphosphate in the pool periodically to reduce the amount of calcium coming from the water. Just how often "periodically" is depends on your local water and can best be determined by local pool experts who have dealt with the water in your area for years. Your pool dealer or contractor can most likely prescribe an effective maintenance program for you.

SOLAR POOL HEATING

A properly engineered and installed solar heating system will keep the temperature of your pool water at whatever level you desire at literally no extra operating cost. That's the good news. The bad news is that the installation of a solar system is expensive, and in many locales the building code demands that with it you must also have a full-blown backup heater that operates on gas, oil, or electricity. Nevertheless, solar is gaining considerable acceptance, particularly in colder regions of the country, and without question it is a viable alternative to standard, energy-consuming heaters.

HOW SOLAR WORKS

In order to heat your swimming pool with a standard solar pool heating array of collectors, you must have an appropriate amount of roof or lawn space to aim the collectors in a true south direction. The collectors *must* face true (not magnetic) south so they can receive sunlight throughout the daylight hours. They must also be angled toward the sun at a degree that is plus or minus 10° of whatever their latitude happens to be.

Since the pool is actually an open storage tank of water, and since that tank is warmed considerably by the sun beating down on it (no matter how weak the sun may be), the temperature of the water rarely needs to be raised more than a few degrees. Consequently, the pool collectors are comparatively inexpensive black rubber or plastic sheets that have no insulation and no glazing over them. Moreover, the pipes servicing the collectors can be PVC plastic, which is considerably less expensive than the copper piping needed to solar heat a hot tub or spa, or the potable water for a home. The trade-off for using

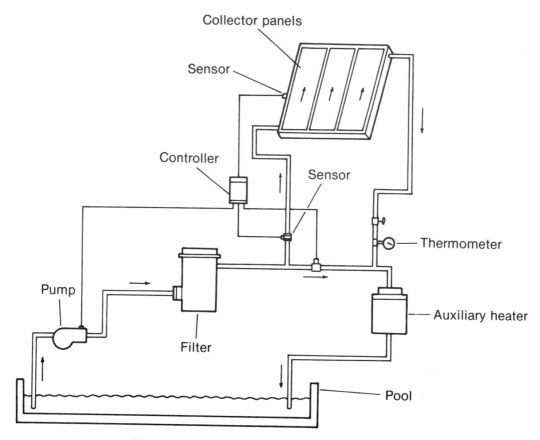

Collector panels

Sensor

Controller

Sensor

Thermometer

Pump

Filter

Auxiliary heater

Pool

The schematic for a typical solar pool heating system.

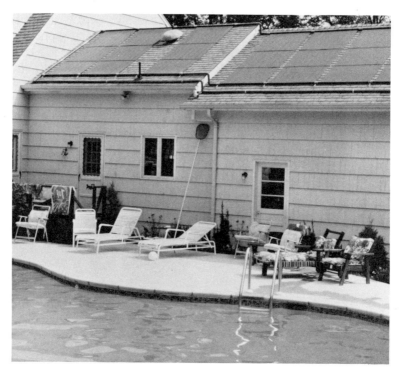

Solar roof collectors for heating a pool.

low-budget pool collectors is that you need a considerable amount of roof space. A 29,000-gallon pool, for example, will require some 512 square feet of collector area, which would be divided into about sixteen panels and would cover a considerable amount of your roof. In general the collector area should be between 50 and 75 percent of the square footage of your pool, unless you plan to use the pool during the coldest months of the year. In that case, the panel area should equal the surface area of the pool.

In some instances, it is possible to use glazed collectors, which will generate hotter water faster, and with considerably fewer panels. However, as soon as you get into higher water temperatures, you have to use copper piping and you have to be careful not to generate so much heat that it has an adverse effect on the chemicals you are putting in your pool water.

You can mount your collectors in any number of ways—on a roof, or tie them to a fence, or lay them out on earth mounds—so long as they are higher than the pool and can be drained in the event of freezing weather. Since you are dealing with unglazed, uninsulated, and frameless pieces of rubber or plastic, they can be held in place in any manner you wish so long as they are supported by some kind of flat surface and held in place in such a way that during their expansion and contraction they do not rub against anything that will wear a hole through the material.

SOLAR CONTROLS

A normal solar heating system involves some complicated controls, including pumps, valves, and a differential thermostat. None of that is absolutely necessary with a pool heating system. The water from the pool is pumped by the filter pump through a network of 3″ PVC pipes, which run under the collector panels and back again. As long as you are running your filter, the water will also be heated, all of which is fine if the sun is shining. If the sun is not shining, or if the pool water is colder than the temperature of the collector panels, and you turn on your filter, you will be in the process of cooling the water in the pool. Consequently, there should be thermostatically controlled diverter valves in the solar pipes that automatically close the pipes to any pool water whenever the temperature of the col-

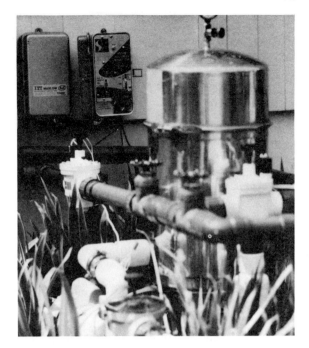

Pool collectors can be serviced by plastic piping.

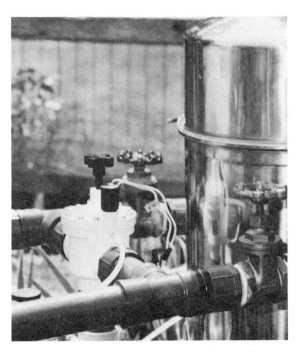

A solar heating system can be run by the pool's standard pump.

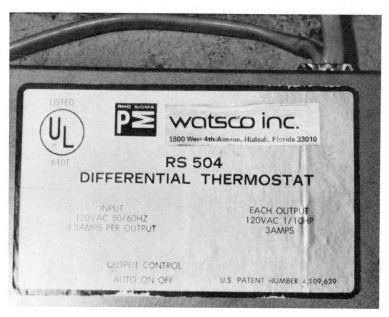

A solar heating system differential thermostat reads the temperature of the water in the pool and at the collectors simultaneously.

lectors is lower than the temperature of the pool water. The control unit need not be elaborate or even expensive, but it should have heat sensors positioned in the pool and at the collector panels and be wired to an electrically operated diverter valve.

A solar pool heating system can cost as much as $3,000 to install, but from then on your only operating costs are for the electricity needed to run the filter pump. Since you must run the filter anyway, you can really only attribute part of the pump costs to heating your water. However, many building codes demand that you must have a standard fossil-fuel heater incorporated into any solar heating system to act as a stand-by in case you want to heat your pool at night, or during very cold, sunless days. In other words, if you live in an area where the building code demands that you have a backup heater for your solar heating system, you are confronted with a double expense which could make incorporating a solar array cost-inefficient.

CHAPTER SIX

Getting Around Your Pool

Whether your pool is aboveground or in-ground, indoors or out, it amounts to a hole in your property which you will presumably fill with water. A hole in your property all by itself can be amazingly unattractive unless you develop a mini-environment around it. And that is where landscaping and things like fences, decks, and cabanas come into your life. You can, in fact, spend more time and effort developing an attractive environment for your pool than you committed to installing the pool itself. Most difficult of all, there are no cut-and-dried rules to follow when you are sprucing up the area around your pool, only some general guidelines that can be considered.

Normally, the landscaping around a pool is not the responsibility of the contractor who built the pool, so often the decking must be relegated to either a different contractor or yourself. Similarly, fences, cabanas, and screen houses are usually separate construction projects that a pool contractor does not become involved in. Nevertheless, all of the elements that create an environment around your pool must be considered at the time you are planning the installation of the pool itself, even if their specific design and con-

struction changes from your original plans when you get around to completing them.

DECKS

The immediate area around your pool is normally at least a 3′ wide concrete walkway. It need not be concrete; it could be a wooden deck. Or the deck might begin at the edge of the walkway and extend out in one, two, or in all directions from the pool, perhaps as far as the limits of your property or the side of the house.

If you do not install a deck, you are subjecting yourself to the possibility of grass cuttings and soil from the yard settling on the surface of the pool water, so decks have a practical advantage as well as some aesthetic ones. They need not, of course, cover every inch of yard space around your pool, and they need not be wooden in construction. You could use flagstones, or concrete slabs, brick, or some other durable material. While all of the materials other than wood that you might use will be placed on or in the ground, wooden decks must be supported above the ground by some means that is durable and more or less impervious to rot.

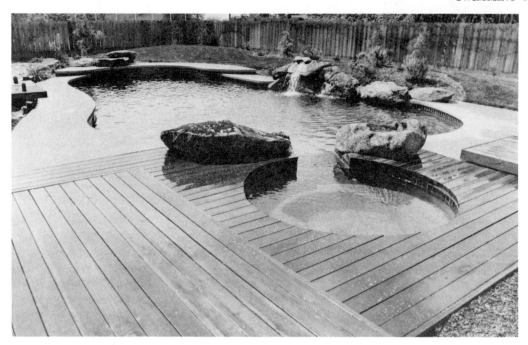

Wood may be the most popular decking material.

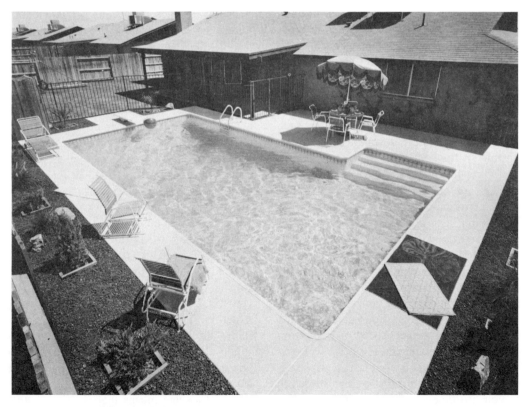

Most pools have at least a 3′ wide deck around their perimeters.

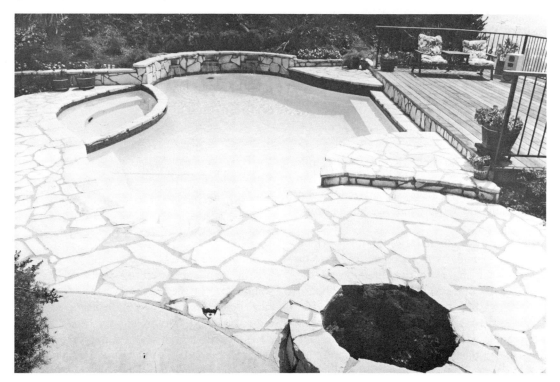

The deck can be made of concrete, flagstone, brick, wood, or any durable, weather-proof material.

There are five basic steps to constructing a wooden deck:

1. Layout and survey of the site, plus measuring for the materials needed.
2. Selecting and ordering all of the required materials.
3. Placing the foundation and ground sheets.
4. Construction of the deck itself.
5. Treating the deck surface.

One of the best things about a wooden deck is that you can design it to suit just about any space. You can tailor it around the side of your house. It can be built at varying levels to blend in with family activities as well as overcome uneven terrain. Wooden decks are about the only way you can give yourself some level outdoor living areas if you happen to be perched on a hillside. On the other hand, if your property is flat, a low-level wooden deck will provide a nonreflective, resilient surface, as opposed to the unforgiving and reflective qualities of concrete or paving stones.

Most pool decks are attached to the side of the house at some point to provide easy access, as well as a partial support, for the decking itself. A low-level deck can be held up by concrete piers or short, closely set together posts, or 4″ × 5″ logs known as landscaping timbers. High-level decks need to be supported by the fewest possible vertical members so that the view of the underside of the deck is not something akin to looking at a stand of pine trees. Each of the supporting posts must, of course, be placed on a concrete footing and usually a heavier deck structure and stronger railings are in order with high decks. Otherwise, the same general rules to ensure a solid deck are applied to both high and low decks.

PLANNING A DECK

No matter what shape or size your deck assumes, it will have to be constructed according to a variety of allowable spans for your decking, joists, and beams, but these depend on the size, grade, and spacing of the framing members. When you plan your deck, check your local building code to be certain you meet all of its requirements.

The Structure

The top of a deck is known as the decking, and it consists of 2″ nominal boards, usually redwood. The most common sizes are 2″ × 4″ and 2″ × 6″ boards that span no more than 24″ on center (o.c.). While redwood is preferred because it has the highest resistance to decay of any wood, you can use specially treated fir, pine, cedar, or western larch.

The decking rests on a series of joists which are 2″ nominal lumber spaced either 16″ o.c. or 24″ o.c. at right angles to the direction of the deck boards. In other words, each deck board crosses over two or more joists and is attached to them. The joists can only be certain lengths, according to their size and type of wood, and the spacing between them. Even at that, some building codes require cross or lateral bracing in-

stalled between the joists to ensure they will not tilt over. In general, the recommended joist spans are:

Nominal Size	Maximum Span
16″ spacing	
2″ × 6″	8′
2″ × 8″	10′
2″ × 10″	13′
24″ spacing	
2″ × 6″	7′
2″ × 8″	8′
2″ × 10″	10′

Beams are used to support the joists, and these are in turn supported by posts or footings of some type. In the case of very level terrain you can sometimes get away with just placing beams on the ground. Beams should be as large as is necessary to minimize the number of posts and footings needed to support the deck and typically are made of 4″ nominal lumber that is 6″, 8″, or

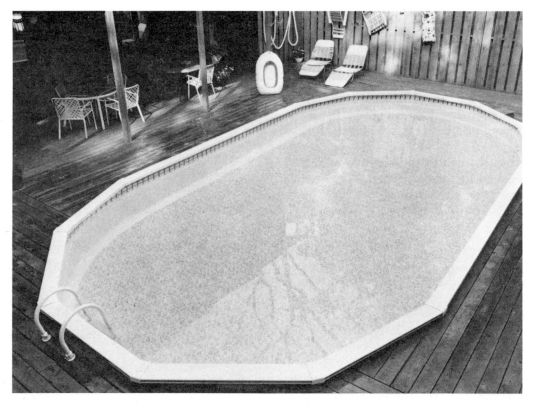

Most wooden decks are attached to the side of the house.

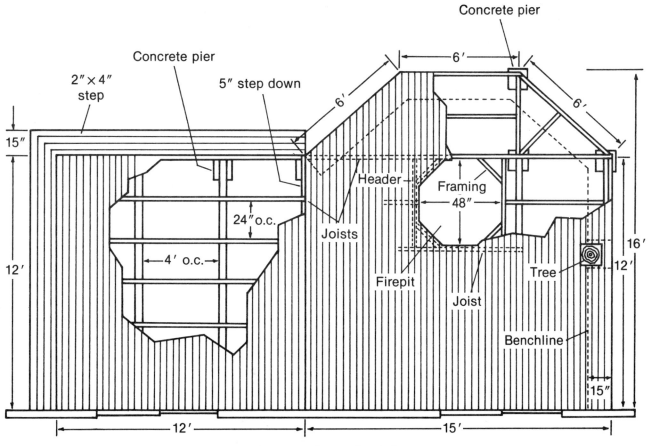

Anatomy of a wooden deck.

10″ wide. If 4″ wood is unavailable, most building codes will allow you to bolt together two pieces of 2″ nominal wood. You can use either bolts or lag screws, but not nails. Again, the span, or the length between supports, of a beam is a function of the dimension of the beams you use:

Beam Size	Width of Deck			
	6′	8′	10′	12′
	Span	Span	Span	Span
4″ × 6″	6′6″	6′	5′	4′
	4′6″	4′	3′6″	3′
4″ × 8″	9′	8′	7′	6′
	6′	5′	4′6″	4′
4″ × 10″	11′6″	10′	8′6″	7′6″
	7′6″	6′6″	6′	5′6″

The *posts* that support the beams are commonly 4″ × 4″, 4″ × 6″, and 6″ × 6″ nominal, depending on the span and spacing of the beams, the load they must support, and the height, as well as the spacing, of the posts themselves. Obviously, if your deck is two stories in the air, your posts ought to be larger and more numerous than if you are laying a ground-level deck. When the deck is fastened to the side of your house, it is usually rigid enough to eliminate the need for bracing between the posts that support it. But if you are erecting a free-standing deck around the edge of an on-ground swimming pool, the posts should have ample cross bracing to keep the structure rigid. The posts must also rest on concrete footings. However, a low-level deck need only be supported on concrete blocks or precast footings.

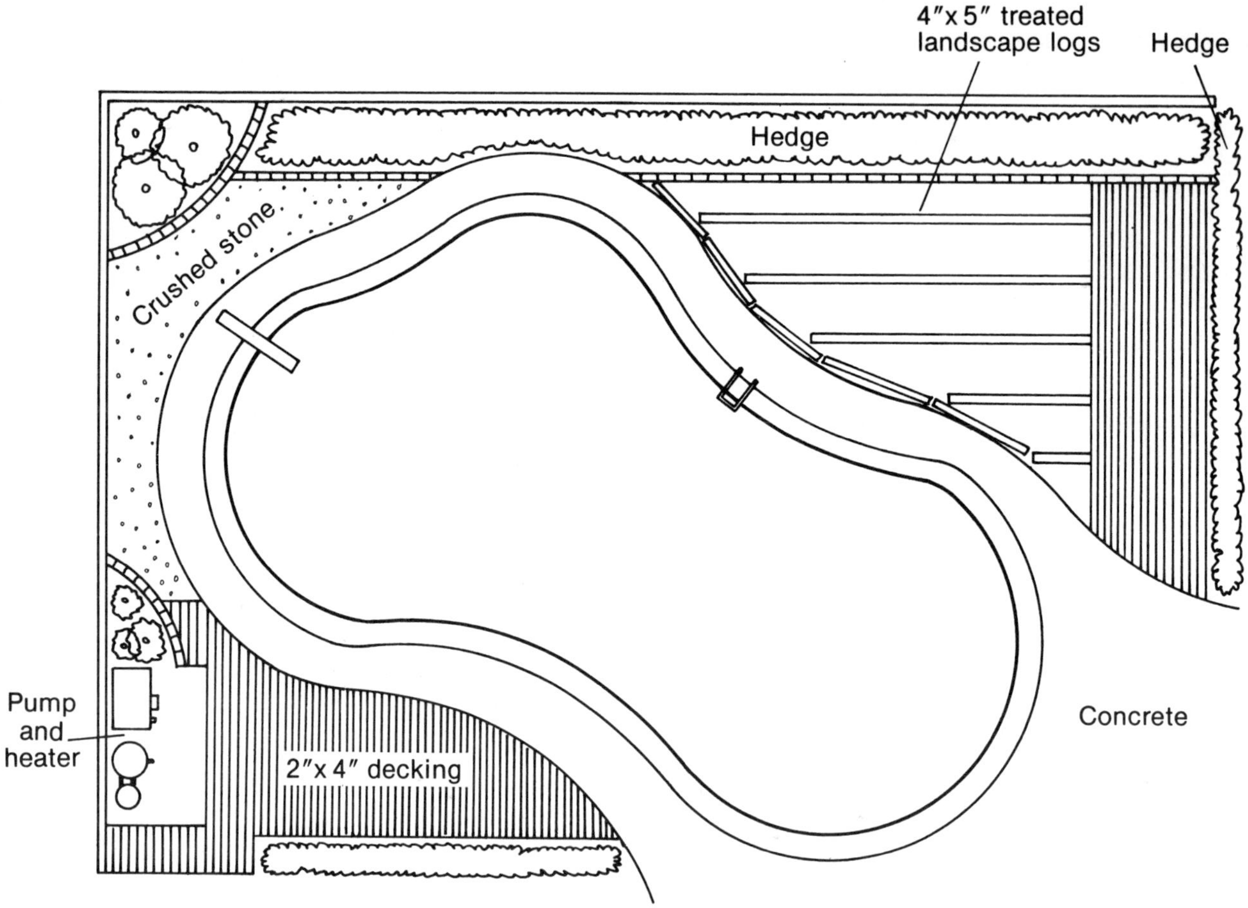

4"x 5" treated landscape logs

Hedge

Hedge

Crushed stone

Concrete

Pump and heater

2"x 4" decking

Anatomy of a ground-level pool deck.

PREPARING THE SITE

The site preparation for a deck is considerably less expensive and less work than it is for a swimming pool. Even if the site is steep, you are not confronted with horrendous earth-moving problems, simply because you do not have to level the ground. You need only be certain there is enough of a grade in the deck to provide adequate runoff of water away from your pool.

Once you have measured the perimeters of your deck, and driven stakes into the ground at each corner, determine where each of the footings will be located and dig holes for the concrete, if the deck is to stand on footings. If you are constructing a low-level deck that ends at the edge of the pool walkway, you can use landscaping logs which have been creosoted or otherwise specially treated to resist decay. The landscaping logs are typically pine and they *must* be properly treated to withstand the dampness of the earth surrounding them.

LAYING LANDSCAPING LOGS

Dig a trench along the walkway surrounding your pool and along whatever stake lines you have placed in the ground to define the outer edges of the deck. A string should be tied tautly between each of your stakes to give you the exact perimeters of the deck, so you can follow them with your trench. The trench should be wide enough and deep enough to contain the logs. Presuming you want the edge of the finished decking to be flush with the surface of the pool walkway, you will have to bury the logs so they are exactly 1⅝" *below* the walkway surface (1⅝" is the real thickness of a 2" nominal deck board). Place the logs around the pool edge first, cutting them so they fit close to the contours of the pool. Then work outward to the outlying edges of the deck, tamping each log down in the trench and making certain they are all leveled. Once you have laid the perimeter logs, place more logs between the edges so they are always 24" o.c. in all directions. The decking should never be asked to span more than 2′ in any direction and the logs should all be laid in the direction that is at right angles to the way your decking will be laid.

Use a 4′ level to keep the logs level and spread dirt from the trenches under and between the logs to keep them firmly in place. The best way of determining the depth of the logs in relation to the surface of the pool walk is to lay a length of your decking board on top of the perimeter logs and make sure it is flush with the concrete walkway.

CONTROLLING GROWTH

Weeds growing beneath any low deck can lead to a high moisture content in the wood members and cause decay, even when the wood has been well treated. Consequently, you must inhibit plant growth under the deck. You can do this by applying a strong weed killer to the plants inside the perimeter of your logs and then laying a sheet of 4- or 6-mil polyethylene or 30-pound asphalt saturated felt over the ground and the logs, allowing the sheeting to sag between the wood to prevent it from tearing. Be certain the plastic sheeting covers every inch of ground. Rain water will, of course, run off the deck and down between the 2″ × 4″ deck boards. If you cannot angle the

plastic or cause furrows in it so that the surface water will run off under the deck, punch a few holes in the plastic to allow some water to escape back into the ground.

FOOTINGS

Decks that must stand a few inches or several feet above the ground require footings, and often footings and posts, to support their beams. In its simplest form, the bottom of a treated post and the friction of the earth around the post will transfer the weight of the deck to the ground. More commonly, concrete is used as a footing to support the post.

The depth of your footings below ground level can vary from 3′ to 5′, depending on the height of the post and the amount of load it must bear. If you live in a warm climate, the footings may be as shallow as 2′ or 3′. In the northern regions, the footing must be placed below the frost line, which means it could be as much as 4′ or 5′ deep. You can best determine the required depth of your footings by checking with your local building code.

Concrete footings are normally used with treated posts and the minimal dimensions of the poured concrete should be 12″ × 12″ × 8″. When you have dug your post holes to the

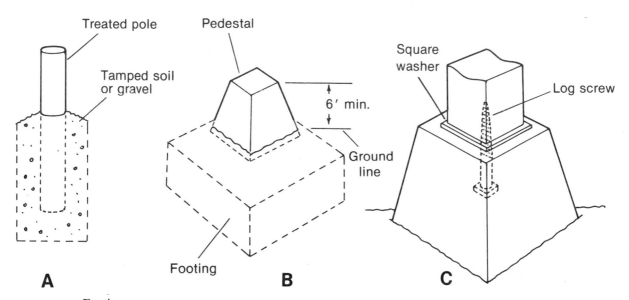

Footings.
A) The easiest and least reliable footing is to sink a treated pole in well-tamped gravel or dirt.
B) Concrete footing pedestals should be at least 6″ higher than grade level.
C) The metal washer placed under the post prevents it from decaying from moisture forming on the concrete.

proper depth, and assuming the hole is 1' square, you then pour 8" of concrete into the bottom of the hole. When the concrete has cured (in about a week) you can then stand the posts on their footings and fill the hole around them with well-tamped soil. Alternatively, you can stand the post in the hole and fill concrete around it almost to ground level.

In situations where you prefer to keep the bottom of the poles aboveground so they will be exposed to the weather but not the ground, you can construct a pier-type pedestal on top of the footings. The footing is poured and then a cone of concrete is built on top of that. The cone is actually a small four-sided pyramid that should end at least 6" above grade level. Its top should be only slightly larger than the size of the post bottoms.

ANCHORING POSTS TO THEIR FOOTINGS

The way you anchor posts to their footings is important, since the connection should be able to resist any lateral movement as well as any uplift stresses that might occur during periods of high winds. These anchorages must also be designed to provide good drainage and prevent decay or damage to the bottom of the post. There are four preferred methods of anchoring posts to their footings and all of them require the use of galvanized metal bolts, screws, and/or fittings.

Small (short) posts can be attached to their footings by inserting a large galvanized lag screw upside down in the top of the footing or pedestal while the concrete is still soft. A square metal washer that is slightly larger than the dimensions of the post bottom is placed over the lag screw and the post is then turned down on the screw until it is secure. The purpose of the metal plate is to prevent any moisture seeping up from the concrete, and providing you are not standing tall members on the screw, it will hold the posts upright without any great difficulty.

A small galvanized, or at least painted, pipe can also be attached to the bottom of a post via a threaded flange. The pipe is sunk in the footing when the concrete is poured and the post is then screwed to the top of the pipe. An alternative version of this arrangement is to use angle irons to attach the post to the pipe, but you will have to position the post in the concrete and brace it

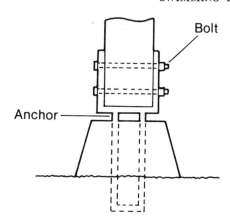

A step-flange is embedded in the concrete and the post can then be bolted between the tynes of the yoke.

to hold it vertical for a week or so until the concrete hardens.

A similar type of post anchor is known as the step-flange, which is essentially a heavy metal bar shaped in the form of a Y. The leg of the flange is buried in the concrete and the post is bolted between the arms of the Y after the concrete footing has set.

BEAM TO POST CONNECTIONS

The beams can be used either to support a system of joists, or to hold the floorboards directly. The reason that beams normally support joists is that they are large and need not be placed close together. So it is less expensive and easier to install a deck if you put the beams as far apart as conditions and the load they will bear allow, and then nail joists over them. But no matter what is immediately attached to them, the beams must also be tied into the posts they rest on.

The beams should be tilted away from the house and the pool at a slope of about 1" for every 10' of their run, to provide a tilt to the deck so that it will shed whatever water lands on it. One way of fastening the beams to each post they cross over is simply to nail 1" × 4" pieces of lumber (exterior grade plywood will do) to two sides of the post, using 8d galvanized nails. Then toenail the cleats to the underside of the beam.

An even better approach is to use angle irons that are large enough to accept galvanized lag screws. Or you can use any of several galvanized metal flanges or straps, which are usually nailed to both the beam and the post with galvanized 8d nails.

When a double post is used you will have something like two 2″ × 6″'s bolted together and a single beam is normally bolted between the two post members. This, however, results in a pair of exposed end-grains in the post boards, which must be protected by wooden cleats nailed to the beam over the ends. If you are using dou-

ble beams, they are normally bolted to either side of the tops of the posts. You can gain a higher load capacity by notching the sides of the post, but in either situation you still end up with the exposed end-grain of the post. Tack a piece of metal flashing or asphalt felt across the beams above the post end as protection against weathering. You do not use the flashing or felt if the post which supports the beam also extends up above the decking to serve as a railing post.

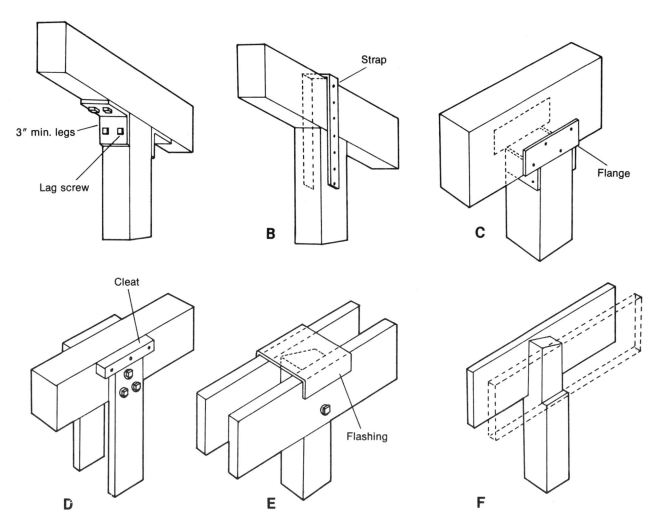

Beam to post connections.
A) Beams and posts can be fastened with metal angles.
B) Straps can also be used to fasten beams and posts.
C) Metal flange fasteners are available at building centers.
D) Cleats must be placed over the exposed end-grains in a double post bolted to a beam.
E) A split beam must have some form of flashing over the post to protect its end-grain.
F) By notching the top of the post, you will gain a better load-bearing construction.

CONNECTING TO THE HOUSE

Many of the decks that are built around swimming pools also connect to the house at some point, usually somewhere near a patio door. You cannot just stop next to the house, but must make a specific connection with the building. The connection is normally made at the beam or joist level using metal hangers, wood ledgers, or angle irons, although in some cases you may be able to utilize the top of the masonry foundation wall (see below). However you work out your hookup, try to do it in such a way that the top of the deck boards resides just under the sill of any doors opening onto the deck. This will give you protection from rain runoff as well as an easy access to the deck.

If the beams are perpendicular to the house, they can often be fastened to the joist header nailed to the sill of the foundation by attaching metal hangers. Or you can bolt or screw a 2″ × 8″ or 2″ × 10″ board to the house framing, and then hang your beams from that, using commercial hangers. You can also anchor a 2″ × 8″ or 2″ × 10″ ledger to the floor framing or masonry wall with expansion plugs and lag screws, and then nail the beam ends to its top. The difference between attaching beams and joists to the house is merely a matter of the size of the metal hangers you use.

BRACING

When you are building a deck across a sloping or an uneven site, or around an on-ground swimming pool, you may wind up with some posts that are several feet high, in which case you will have to provide bracing to give them lateral stability. If the deck is a free-standing unit (such as around an on-ground swimming pool), brace along each side of the unit. You can use 2″ × 4″'s if the braces are no longer than 8′; any lengths over that should be 2″ × 6″'s. The accepted method of attachment is to use either bolts or lag screws to tie the braces into each post they touch.

Bracing is rarely, if ever, horizontal, but is usually arranged so that it forms a series of triangles with the vertical posts. One system of bracing calls for a series of "W"'s in which every other post accepts the high ends of the braces which rise from the bottoms of the two adjacent posts. You can also create a series of "X"'s when the height of the post is unusually high. In this instance, each X is formed between posts with the ends of the braces bolted to the posts and to each other at the point they cross in the center. Normally, X bracing is required only at every other bay, or spacing, between the posts.

With posts that are between 5′ and 7′ high, a plywood gusset or short braces cut from 2″ nominal lumber are sufficient. The plywood gussets are triangles cut from ¾″ exterior grade plywood and nailed to both sides of the top of the post and the beam it holds. The top edges of the plywood must be protected by a header or an edge to protect the end-grain. Nail the gussets to the post and beam with 10d galvanized nails spaced every few inches.

A partial brace made from 2″ × 4″ lumber is

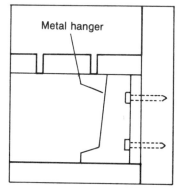 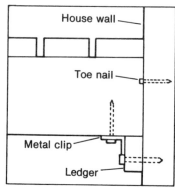

Connecting to the house.
A) You can attach a 2″ × 8″ or 2″ × 10″ ledger to the side of the house with lag screws and then connect beams or joists to it using metal hangers.
B) You can also rest the deck structure on a ledger and secure your connections with metal angles.

Bracing.

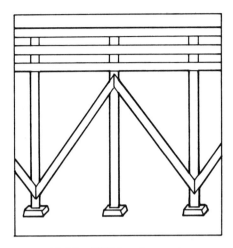

A) The "W" bracing system.

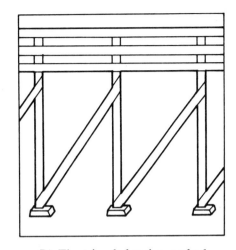

B) The triangle bracing method.

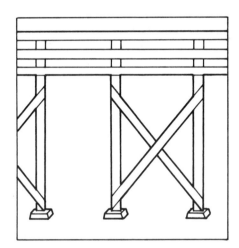

C) The "X" bracing system.

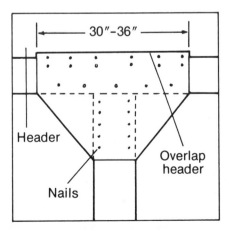

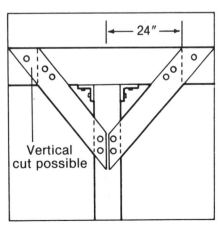

Gussets and braces.
A) Plywood gussets should be made of ¾″ exterior-grade plywood.
B) Short braces can be 1″ and 2″ nominal lumber; be sure to cut the ends so they are vertical or are amply protected from the weather.

secured to the beam and the post with galvanized lag screws or bolts. Again you have to protect the end-grains, either by cutting the ends of the brace at a vertical angle, or by positioning a framing member or deck boards over the ends. The partial bracing extends from the top of the beam a foot or two down the side of the posts.

JOISTS TO BEAMS

When the beams are spaced either 16″, 24″, or conceivably as much as 48″ apart, you can attach 2″ × 4″ decking directly to them without using intermediate joists. However, if the beams are more than 4′ apart, a system of supporting joists must be placed at right angles over them (see below). The joists should be stood on edge across the beams and spaced every 16″ o.c. or 24″ o.c. The nominal dimensions of the joists depends on their span, as shown in the chart below:

Joist Size	Maximum Span
1″ × 4″	16″
2″ × 4″, laid flat	36″
2″ × 6″, laid flat	42″
2″ × 3″, laid on edge	72″
2″ × 4″, laid on edge	120″

Any joist that bears directly on a beam can be toenailed into the beam using two 10d galvanized nails on each side. If you live in a high-wind area, you may want to use 24- to 26-gauge galvanized strapping with 1″ galvanized roofing nails at each joint as added support.

If there is to be a header nailed across the ends of the joists, situate it so that it extends beyond the beams by half an inch to provide a drip edge.

LAYING DECK BOARDS

Deck boards are face-nailed or screwed to every beam or joist that they cross. Both nails and screws must be countersunk slightly below the surface of the board, and the boards should be spaced ⅛″ apart to allow for expansion and water runoff.

When your deck ends at the concrete walkway around a swimming pool, your particular concern is to make the ends of each deck board fit snugly against the concrete curbing. The boards should, of course, lay perpendicular across the beams buried in the ground beside the pool. Always work with the longest spans first so that any short ends that must be cut from the boards can be used in narrower parts of the deck to minimize waste. Measure and cut each piece so that it will fit precisely against the concrete and also end at the center line of one of the beams. In

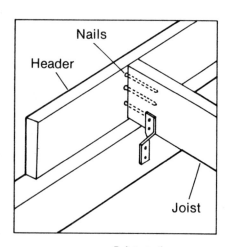 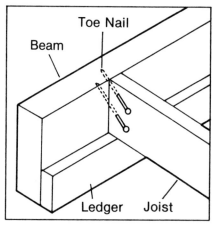 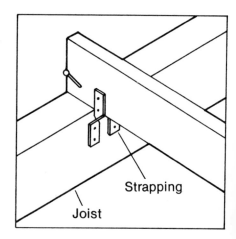

Joists to beams.
A) When you use a header joist, nail into the end of each joist, or use a twist strap.
B) If a joist lands between beams, toenail into the beam and support the joist with a ledger.
C) Joists may also be toenailed to the top of a beam and then strengthened with metal straps.

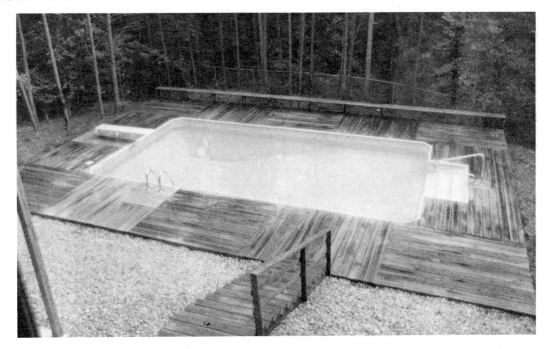

The ends of a ground-level deck must be flush with the side of the pool, or the edge of its concrete apron.

order to make the proper cuts in the pool end of the boards, lay each board over the cement and mark its sides at the point it crosses over the cement, then draw a guideline between your markings and cut off the end. You can maintain an even spacing between boards by tacking a common nail against the previous board at each of its ends. The nail heads should be just below the surface of the previously laid 2″ × 4″ so they can keep the next board properly spaced. The spacer nails can be pulled as soon as the next board has been nailed in place. Always work from the pool edge back across your beams, and always make any end to end joints between boards over a beam so that both board ends can be properly nailed in place.

RAILINGS

With free-standing decks around on-ground pools, or with any deck that is more than a foot or two above ground level, you will want to include a system of balusters or rail posts for protection. The critical members of the baluster system are, in reality, posts that have been extended above the level of the deck to whatever height your railing is to be. The railing height can vary from 30″ to 40″ or more if there is a bench or windscreen involved, and the posts that support a 2″ × 4″ horizontal top rail should not be more than 6′ apart. If the top rail is a 2″ × 6″ board, the posts can be as much as 8′ apart.

When you are unable to extend the posts above the deck, you may be able to attach the rail posts to a joist or beam. Rail posts are normally constructed from pieces of 2″ × 6″ for spans of less than 4′, or 2″ × 8‴s for spans of 4′ to 6′, and from 2″ × 6‴s or 3″ × 8‴s for 6′ to 8′ spans. Bolt each post to the edge beam with two bolts spaced as far apart as you can reasonably get them without splitting any of the wood.

The ends of beams or joists under the edge of your deck can also be used to support rail posts, but avoid mounting any rail post to the deck boards. Not only will you have a structurally weak railing, but the bottoms of the posts will be in contact with a flat surface that could trap water under the post and produce rapid decay of the wood.

A cap rail across the top of the posts will pro-

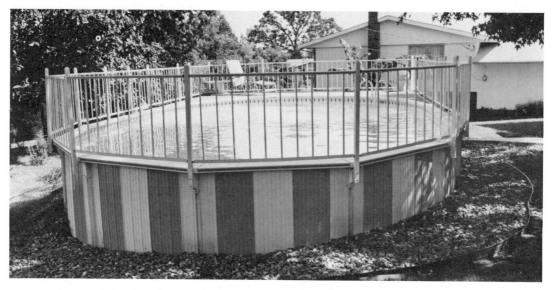

Any pool that is more than 2′ aboveground should have a protective railing around it.

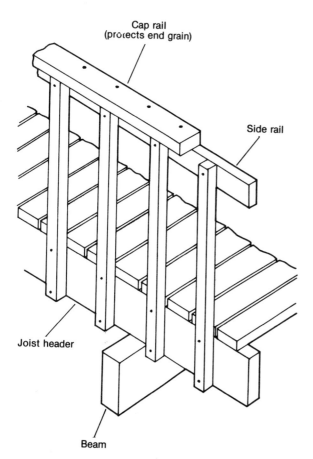

Anatomy of a typical deck railing.

tect their end-grains from water damage, but the railing will be structurally sounder if you also bolt a side rail across the face of the posts to tie them together. The side, or face, rail can be directly under the top of the posts and/or partway between the decking and the rail cap.

STAIRWAYS

The stairways needed to provide access to and from a deck are constructed in much the same manner as any indoor stairway except that you must be careful to avoid any moisture traps under the exposed end-grains that could cause more rapid than normal decay. Stairways can be one- or two-step affairs that lead from deck level to deck level, or they can be several steps that get you up to the top of an on-ground pool. In any case, the steps are held in place by 2″ × 10″ or 2″ × 12″ stringers placed not more than 3′ apart. The stringers must be secured to the deck framing (not the deck boards) and can rest on a ledger or by the extension of a pair of beams or joists. The preferred method of tying stringers to the framing is with a ledger nailed to the framing and metal hangers, unless the extension of a joist or beam is situated so that the stringers can be bolted to it.

Stringers.

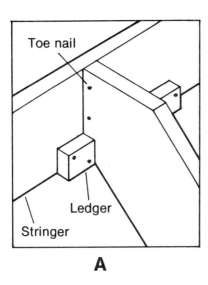

A

A) Stair stringers can be hung from a small ledger.

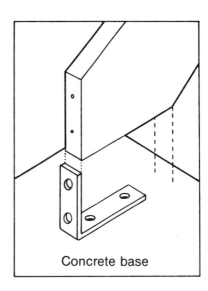

Concrete base

If the bottom of the stair stringer is to touch concrete, protect the wood with an angle iron.

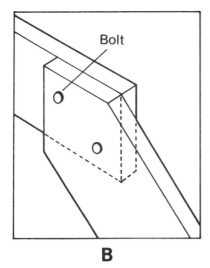

B

B) If you have the end of a joist or beam to work with, bolt the stair stringers to it.

The bottom of the stringers must also be anchored to a solid base and isolated from any source of moisture. If you are going from deck to deck, you can simply nail the bottom of the stringers to the decking. But if the stairway ends at the ground, it should be rested on a concrete footing, sloped for drainage, and each stringer secured by metal angles that are thick enough to keep the wood off the concrete.

The stringers are notched to accept the stair treads, and the relationship of the tread width to its rise (height) is important both for the sake of safety and in determining the number of steps required. The rise of each step in inches multiplied by the width of the tread in inches should equal between 72″ and 75″. For example, if the rise is 8″ and the tread is 9″ wide, 8″ × 9″ = 72″.

Stair treads are usually supported by dadoes, or notches cut in the stringers. However, the notches create an exposed end-grain in the vertical cut, plus the end-grains of both ends of each tread. A more suitable approach is to nail 2″ × 3″ or 2″ × 4″ cleats to the insides of the stringers to support the treads (see p. 88). An even better method, which will avoid water traps, is to bolt 2″ × 4″ ledgers to the stringers and extend them to support the treads. The ends of the ledgers should be angled slightly inward to avoid water collecting on them.

On high stairways with one or both sides unsupported, there should be a system of railings. These are constructed in the same manner as deck railings; in fact, for the sake of visual compatibility, they should be made in the exact manner as your deck rails.

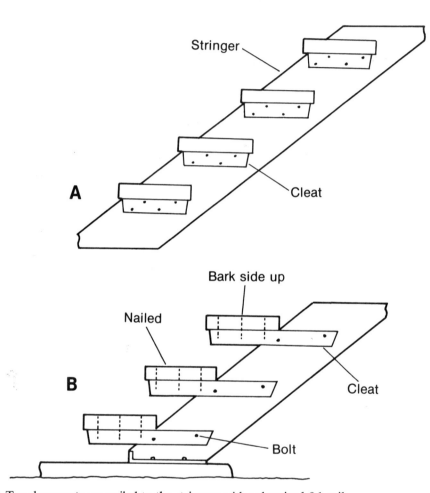

A) Tread supports are nailed to the stringers with galvanized 8d nails.
B) The bolted cleat approach is considered preferable for deck stair construction. Be sure to cut all exposed grain ends vertically.

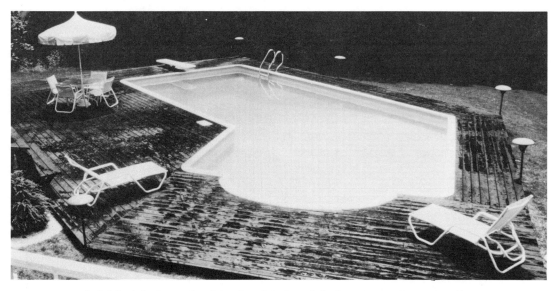

A finished deck can be stained, painted, or left alone to weather naturally.

DECK FINISHING

The final step in constructing a deck is to give it a surface treatment. You can use any type of oil stain or paint, or for that matter allow the treated wood to weather a natural gray. Stains are available in all tints, and they will never cause the deck surface to become slippery the way paint will. All stains soak into the dry wood and help its resistance to decay; the transparent ones allow the wood grain to show through, which many people find attractive.

FENCES

A fence or windscreen can serve your pool in many ways. It can establish a privacy, shielding you from passers-by and neighbors alike as you use your pool. It can add color and décor that extend the atmosphere around your pool. It can block out eyesores and establish the boundary lines of your property, and can be used to divide the activity areas in your yard. A fence may also be mandated by your local building code as a safety requirement to protect children and unwary strangers from falling into the water when it is unattended. A fence, if it is placed against the prevailing breezes, can push the wind up above the surface of the water, reducing the amount of surface evaporation and making an otherwise cool day still comfortable for swimming.

PLANNING A FENCE

Your local statutes regarding pool fences are likely to be very specific as far as their setbacks from the property line, as well as the type and size they must be. Nevertheless, any fence intended for shelter from the wind and/or sun should be carefully designed. For example, a fence with adjustable louvers (either horizontal or vertical) can be opened to allow gentle solar rays through it, then closed when the heat becomes too intense. This same design can, of course, be used to control the breezes playing over your pool. If, for example, a strong, cold north wind is blowing, you can close the louvers and force the wind to rise well above the pool surface. Or you can open them to allow a gentle southerly breeze to warm the pool area. The louver panels can be made of wood as well as colored plastic or fiberglass.

In considering fences, you must first take into account the contour of the land. Designs that require straight runs, that is paneled or picket fence types, are not particularly suited for hilly ground. A rambling or step-down fence is more adaptable for a sloped area. And never overlook the appearance of the fence in terms of your neighborhood and the architecture of your house.

Although the term "fence" normally implies a wooden or sometimes metal or plastic structure, you may discover that your specific needs are

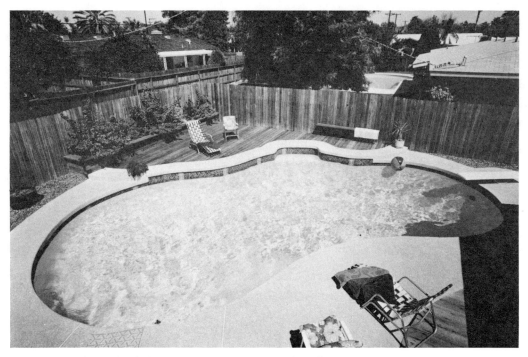

A fence or windscreen can provide several benefits for any pool.

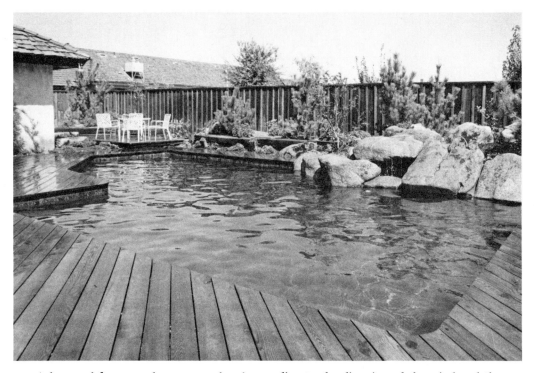

A louvered fence can be open or closed according to the direction of the wind and the temperature.

best met by brick, stone, or decorative concrete block.

FENCE POSTS

Wooden fences usually rely on vertical posts for their stability. The one exception to that rule is a zigzag fence, which needs posts only to anchor it to the ground. Posts can range in dimension from 2″ × 4‴s, 3″ × 3‴s, to 4″ × 4‴s and 3″ to 6″ logs, and as a rule, one third of their total length is below ground. Thus, if you were erecting a 6′ high fence, the length of its posts would be 9′.

The first point to be considered with fence posts is their spacing. Prebuilt fences typically come in 6′ or 8′ lengths, which are supported at each end by a post, but check the type you are buying before you start erecting posts, as some preformed products come in odd lengths. If you are constructing your own fence, you have the advantage of placing your posts as far apart as you wish, although 8′ on center is the most common spacing. You have to be reasonable about the distances between your posts. For example, suppose you had a fence that was 33′ long. If the posts are 8′ apart, you will have five posts 8′ apart and a 1′ section left over. You might do better to split the extra foot among all of the sections and place the posts 8′3″ apart or put up

seven posts spaced every 5′6″. You also need to take into consideration the width of gates and make allowances for where they will be placed in the fence.

Once you have determined your property boundaries and setbacks (by reading your local building code), mark off your fence using a 50- or 100-foot tape measure or string. Mark the location of each post hole by driving stakes into the ground. The post holes can be dug with a square-end spade, but a more serviceable tool is a post-hole digger, which can usually be rented. Auger-type post-hole diggers are best for rock-free soil; clam-shell diggers are preferred if you are likely to encounter a lot of rocks and stones.

Dig each hole 4″ deeper than the required depth of the post and fill the bottom of the holes with a 4″ layer of gravel to guarantee proper drainage away from the bottoms of the posts. The diameter of the hole will vary with the size of the post but generally, if the post is to be set in tamped earth, the hole should be twice the diameter of the post. If you are setting the post in concrete, make the hole two and a half times the diameter of the post.

Treat every fence post with liberal coatings of a preservative such as creosote and be particularly sure the bottom and top end-grains are well saturated. If you are setting the posts in tamped

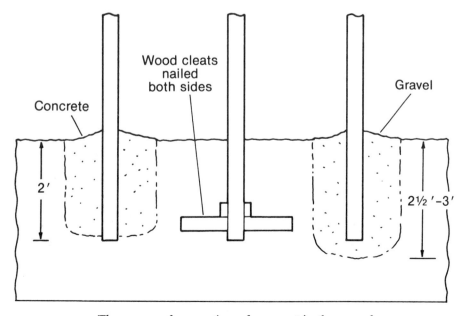

Three ways of supporting a fence post in the ground.

soil or gravel, nail 1″ × 2″ cleats in all directions across the bottom of the post, then place the two end poles in their holes. Run a taut string between the two posts and use a line level to make sure they are properly aligned with each other. Use a carpenter's level to plumb both posts and brace them temporarily with boards nailed to stakes driven into the ground. Now backfill the post holes with earth or gravel, tamping it firmly around the post. Mound the earth slightly around the base of the posts to direct water runoff away from the wood.

The best way to ensure a sturdy fence post is to backfill its hole with concrete. However, make very certain that the bottom of the post is firmly embedded in loose gravel to allow good drainage and is not resting on concrete, where puddles can accumulate and accelerate the rotting of the post bottoms.

Once the two end posts are set, place the intermediate posts, using the string line as your guide for both straightness and height.

BUILDING YOUR FENCE

You can find plans for all kinds of fences in magazines and how-to books devoted to outdoor structures. In general, rails or stringers placed at the top and bottom of the post should be 2″ × 4‴s and the slats that are nailed to them are usually 1″ × 8‴s or 1″ × 10‴s, although they can actually be any width of 1″ stock you choose. Picket fences, for example, are usually 1″ × 3‴s or 1″ × 4‴s. The nails used to assemble your fence should be galvanized or aluminum: 12d or 16d nails are used for attaching rails and 8d's are used with the boards.

You can stain or paint a wooden fence, just as you would a deck.

GATES

One end of every gate hangs free from any support other than the hinges on its opposite side. As a result, the posts that protect a gate must be unusually sturdy, particularly because as part of a moving portion of the fence, they will absorb considerable abuse. It is advisable to set gate posts in concrete, even if the rest of the posts in your fence are placed in tamped soil or gravel. You should also use heavier lumber (4″ × 6‴s

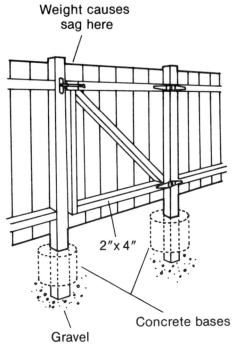

Weight causes sag here

2″ x 4″

Concrete bases

Gravel

Anatomy of a gate.

or 4″ × 4‴s, for example) if the over-all design of the fence permits.

Gates should be wide enough to accommodate at least two people side by side, which means they should be a minimum of 3′ wide. Actually, anything wider than 3′ can make the gate too heavy and cause it to sag from its own weight, pulling at the hinge screws. If the gate opening is more than 3′, consider using two gates. No matter what the width of the gate, the best way of giving it extra strength is to add a diagonal brace (a 2″ × 4″ is good) from the top of the free side to the bottom of the hinge side. And if the gate is unusually heavy, additional bracing should be considered.

The hinges used on gates should be long and heavy and they should be attached with long screws, if not bolts. Leave ½″ clearance at the free side, and be sure there are no obstructions in the way of its swing, and that it does not swing uphill. If the gate is at the top of a stairway leading to a free-standing deck around an on-ground pool, it should have a latch on its inside (the pool side) that can be reached by adults, but not small children.

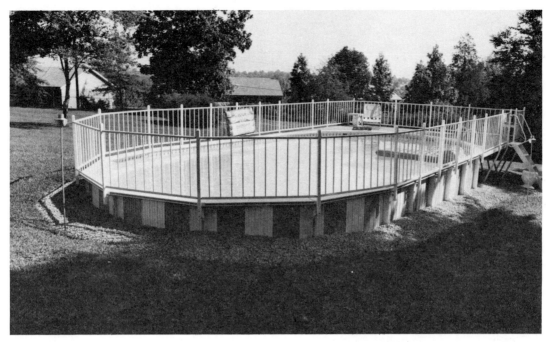

The entranceway at the top of a stairway to an on-ground pool should have a gate with an inside lock that can be worked by adults but not small children.

LANDSCAPING

Your pool, whatever shape it is, however large it might be, and no matter what you have spent to install it, requires some sort of ambience around it. The pool itself can set the tone of how your property will look, but it must be decorated to create a pleasant setting for leisure time activities, just as any indoor room must be decorated. Entertaining friends beside your pool while the space around it is a barren, dusty desert is about as much fun as having a party in a cluttered basement, no matter how terrific a host you might be. In other words, a well-kept lawn, with some carefully located plantings, shrubs, and trees, can make all the difference in the world. The plantings can serve as "room dividers" between various activity areas, to say nothing of functioning as windscreens and sun shades.

NATURAL FORCES

It's your property and you can do what you want with it—up to a point. If you want to lounge around under your own magnolia tree sipping mint juleps, that's fine. But if you live in the state of Maine, you'd better go for pine trees instead, because magnolias can't survive in cold weather. You can't change the weather, either. You can make some allowances for it, and even talk about it a lot, but you can't change it. The most you can do about the weather when you are landscaping is to select trees and shrubs that will thrive in the local temperature ranges with the average rainfall you get in your back yard. If you want to force the issue a little and plant some trees or shrubs that need more water than you normally get during each year, you can install a sprinkling system, but that is about all. If you have strong prevailing winds, you may have to protect some of your young plants and trees with windscreens, but generally your selection of plantings must take into account the topography of your property.

A flat plain can acquire some visual interest if you group your plantings in corners or around specific activity areas (such as your swimming pool). A steep lawn that is hard to mow anyway might be planted with trees or ground cover. Or it might be terraced and planted with shrubs and flowers. It could also be covered by a multi-level

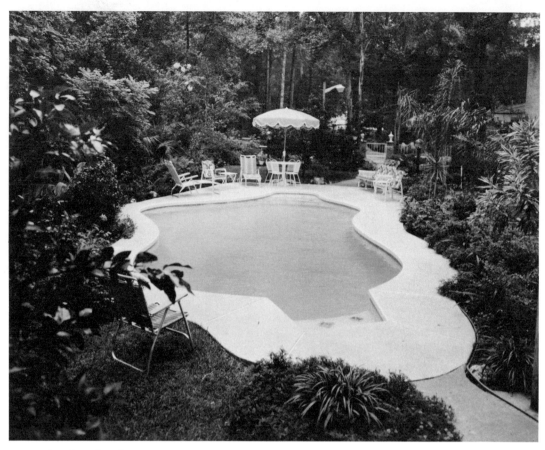

Landscaping has a great deal to do with the pleasurable environment around your pool.

deck. The soil in your back yard is another factor to be considered. Have it tested to determine its pH factor (whether it has too much acid or alkali) so that you have an idea about what minerals must be added to the soil for the kinds of plants you want to grow. Clay, hardpan, or very sandy topsoil may have to be replaced, at least in the areas where you want to grow plantings, so there is a root zone that will permit moisture to soak in, rather than run off, or just stay on the surface of the ground.

HUES

As color is important to interior decoration, so does it control a vital part of your outdoor décor. Green is the restful abundance of nature, and there are many, many shades of it to be found in plantings. Some people use only different shades of green found in the leaves of deciduous trees, broadleaf evergreens, and needle-leaf evergreens. Others add touches of the brilliant as well as subtle colors found in flowering plants to bring a splash of color to their yards all year long. They will plant yellow, white, and violet crocuses that erupt in color while the last vestiges of snow are still on the ground. Then come the daffodils and tulips so early in the spring you are likely to be still wearing a sweater outdoors. From then on there are the flowering ornamental trees with their reds, pinks, and whites, and the roses that can be found in nearly every color imaginable. By mid-summer you can have mimosa, larkspur, zinnias, asters, and petunias. And with the fall, there are the bright red berries of the dogwood (the same folks who brought you flowers during the spring) plus golden rain, crape myrtle, and Chinese dogwood.

You can find all sorts of flowering plants to decorate the space around your pool, but be a little restrained. You can overplant a yard as easily as you can overdecorate a room and create color combinations that clash and take away from the serenity of your pool. Evergreens mixed with flowering plants, particularly around the edges of a deck, can provide some admirable restraint as well as some restful repetition no matter what or where you are landscaping. Restraint should be exercised in the types of plantings you select, as well as their numbers. Plants need room to grow, and too many different types of plants can make your yard look cluttered. By repeating the same plant texture and the same colors, or tones of the same color, in different parts of the yard, you can help to unify your landscaping. But again, don't go overboard. Avoid having plants that are all the same size or texture or color.

TREES

If you have an older home, you probably also have some trees on your property. And unless they are blocking an unusual view, or are diseased, or happen to be standing right in the middle of where you want to put your swimming pool, you would rarely consider cutting them down. But people who move into a new house are usually not as fortunate and must plant their own trees. Unfortunately, transplanting a mature tree is both difficult and expensive, and there is precious little guarantee of the tree living for very long. Which means if you are planting trees around your swimming pool, they will likely be of sapling proportions. You have to use some vision about young trees because what you put in the ground today is not what you will have tomorrow. You can plant practically anything next to your swimming pool if it is a sapling, but ten years from now the root system of those cute lit-

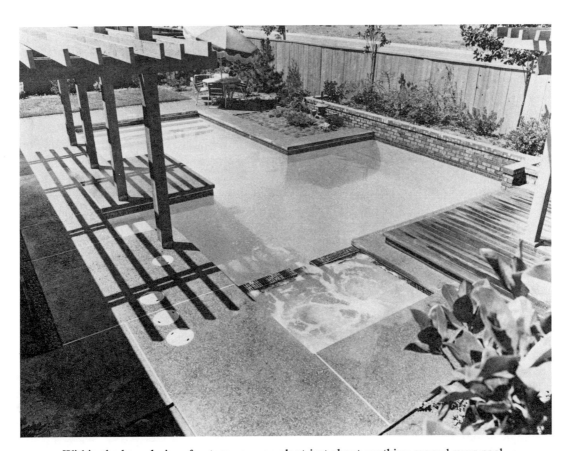

Within the boundaries of nature you can plant just about anything around your pool.

tle sticks in the ground could become so large and powerful that they will begin to break up the sturdiest of concrete pool walls. Today's saplings will not provide a great deal of shade as you paddle about your pool. A few years from now your pool could be completely under foliage all summer, and deluged with leaves in the fall. In other words, if you are planting trees near your swimming pool, be very careful about where you put them and the kind of trees you buy.

It makes sense to adhere to the advice of local landscaping experts when making your tree selection. Here are some general thoughts about trees that you might consider, but the final answers to all of your questions should come from someone who is familiar with your region, its soil and annual rainfall, its climate, and the kinds of trees that will best survive in your particular locale:

Trees are divided into two main classifications, evergreen and deciduous. Evergreens keep their leaves all year long and include such species as pine, fir, spruce, holly, hemlock, and cedar. Deciduous trees shed their leaves in the fall of each year and include all of the fruit trees, oak, larch, hickory, maple, sycamore, and willow. Deciduous trees usually grow faster than evergreens, but that growth rate is affected by the fertility of the soil, rainfall, and the temperature range.

One of the things you have to consider when you pick a tree is whether it can survive the climate where you live. Any tree that is native to your region will obviously be able to live in your back yard. However, there are plenty of species that might be introduced to your yard that could also survive there. If you live in a northern region, you must be careful to make your selection based on cold-hardiness. If you live in a hot, dry area, you can certainly plant any of several alien species, providing you are willing and capable of following specific watering practices. On the other hand, it might be easier to select a drought-resistant species, particularly if water is becoming a precious commodity in your area.

The root systems of willows, elms, poplars, and maples are awesome and have an unending thirst. They force their way in all directions looking for water and have been known to punch their way into sewer lines and clog drainage pipes. Lovely as they are, all of these species should be kept well away from your swimming pool and its underground water lines.

There are many species that have shallow root systems which remain so close to the surface of the ground that they will disrupt walkways or patios, or the skirt around an in-ground swimming pool. The sycamore, for example, has a root system that can easily heave one end of a concrete patio clear out of the ground.

In order to shade a deck or patio near your pool, you might consider one big tree, but a cluster of smaller ones could achieve the same aim a lot faster. As a rule of thumb, shade trees should be planted west and a little south of whatever it is you want to shade. But in no case should you plant any trees so close together that they will grow up to entangle their branches. And don't plant any of those cute little saplings under an overhead power line, either.

FOUNDATION PLANTING

Most homes have partially exposed foundations made of concrete or masonry block. There are often concrete walkways and patios, and once you have installed a pool, there is likely to be more concrete around that as well. While concrete is a durable building material, it can be relatively unattractive if left by itself. So people spend a considerable amount of time, effort, and money decorating their concrete, or just plain hiding it. Low shrubs, hedges, and vines can be used around the foundation of your house, to say nothing of flowers. But most of the plants around your pool and deck should be low-growing varieties. You can use some higher-growing shrubs near the deck areas, provided the decks are well above ground level. You should put low-growing plants along any steps and gateways you may have, to provide a feeling of safe, easy access to the deck or pool.

CABANAS AND SCREEN HOUSES

Cabanas, bathhouses, or similar buildings are ideal addenda to a pool if the pool is well away from the house. They can be any size you wish and include a shower, water closet, lockers, or whatever accommodations you desire. They are also an artful way of hiding the filtering plant.

You can design and build your own structure or purchase prefabricated units that are easily assembled. You can also build a screen house around the pool. The screen might be attached to the side of your house or form a free-standing

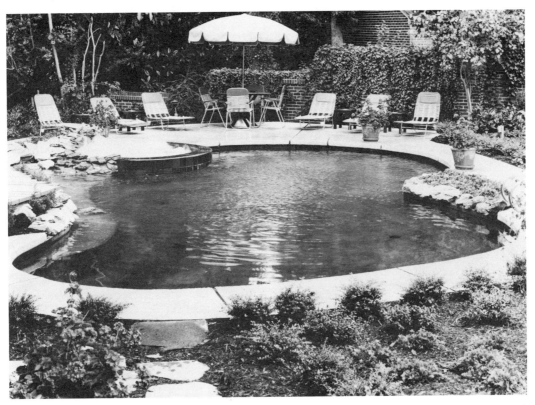

There are all kinds of low plants that can be used around the foundation of your home and ground-level concrete.

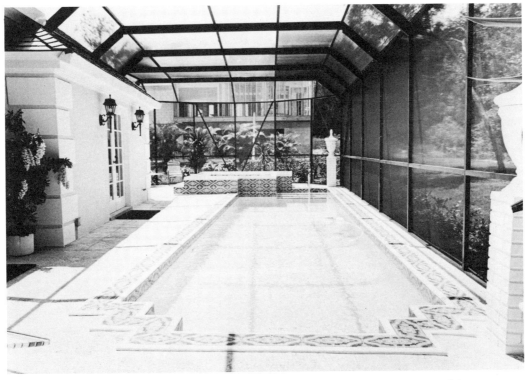

Screen houses are excellent for keeping out bugs and strangers while still giving you the feeling of being in the open.

structure, but in either case the idea is to surround your pool with a screen to keep out bugs and debris, as well as protect neighborhood children from falling into the water. Screen houses are also available in prefabricated form and can be used with metal or fiberglass panels or awnings to give privacy and protection against the sun.

AIR-INFLATED STRUCTURES

With the expansion of residential pools to the colder regions of America has come the air-inflated pool structure. Looking like half a dirigible parked over your pool, the structures are made of tough, durable plastic fabrics which are transparent enough to let in sunlight. The structure is anchored to the walk around the pool, filled with air, and kept rigid by a small electric blower so that it remains sturdy enough to withstand strong winds.

The air structures are used in combination with a heating unit and blower which produce a steady flow of warm, fresh air. The climate inside the air building is totally controllable, so it can be as warm as you wish, but it is recommended that you still have a heater to warm the pool water.

While air-filled pool houses are expensive, they do offer the advantage of extending your swimming season all year around. They also provide protection for the pool throughout the winter as well as keep leaves and other debris out of the water. The units can be inflated in about two hours and then dismantled and folded away for the summer in an easily stored package.

CHAPTER SEVEN

The Care and Maintenance of Pools

If you are one of, or about to be one of, the more than four million Americans who recreate in their own swimming pools, the care and maintenance of your watery playground are of utmost importance. Maintenance may not be much fun, but if you don't do the dirty work on a regular basis, you won't have a pool to play in.

Swimming is one of the most energy-efficient recreations we have, even though the cost of operating a home pool continues to rise in direct proportion to the rising cost of energy. But in order to maintain that energy efficiency there are some little extra steps that must be taken. The National Swimming Pool Institute, which is an industry-supported association of firms involved in the pool industry, offers several suggestions for conserving energy. In summary, the NSPI estimates that if you use a pool cover, perform a regular maintenance program, and carefully regulate the operating times of your filtration, cleaning, and heating systems to coincide with when your pool is in use, you will be able to operate your pool at a cost of less than one dollar a day. *And* you will conserve a considerable amount of energy.

OPERATIONAL MAINTENANCE

There is a simple art to proper pool care. If you organize your time and the procedures properly, it should not require more than an hour or two of your time each week to complete all of the necessary maintenance chores.

POOL COVERS

To begin with, own and use a pool cover. Depending on the climate, a pool cover can represent a 50 to 75 percent saving on heating your pool. The purpose of a cover is to minimize heat loss from the pool surface through evaporation and radiation of the warm water to cooler surrounding air. If you slap a cover over the pool, it helps keep heat in the water and therefore cuts down on the amount of work your heater has to do. As a matter of fact, some types of covers actually raise the pool temperature by increasing the ability of the water to transmit and retain heat from the sun's rays. Don't let the cost of a cover stand in your way, either. A cover can be made to fit any pool and it can be pulled over the

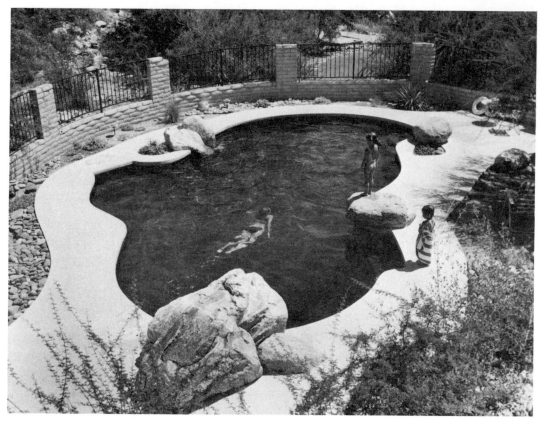

More than 4 million Americans enjoy residential pools each year.

water or removed by one person. If you take care of it, a cover will last for years—and it will reduce your utility bills by at least as much as its purchase price during the first year you own it.

FILTERS

The function of a pool filter is to draw water from the pool continuously, pass it through the filter, and return the purified water to the pool. The water in your pool should always be clear enough so that you can tell whether a dime lying on the bottom of the deep end is heads or tails up. You can run your pump and filter for about six to eight hours every day and keep the water in your pool very clear and extremely sanitary. But the chances are that six to eight hours is more filtration time than you really need. So reduce it.

You can determine the minimum filtration time by gradually shortening your present cycle period until the water turns murky, or until a chemical test that includes a check for disinfectant residual shows an improper balance. At that point, increase the filtration cycle by one half hour and lock your time clock. Lock it, but don't throw away the key. The amount of filtration time needed will be longer during times when the pool is in constant use. So at the beginning or end of the season when the pool is being used less, you can reset the time downward.

Another hint about filtration time: If you live in an area where the utility rates are higher during peak-use periods, set the timer so that your filtration period is before and after the peak periods, and not during them. To do this automatically, you may have to install a second set of trippers on your time clock, but these are neither expensive nor difficult to incorporate.

Just remember that when you are playing the minimum filtration game, you must still run the filter whenever the pool is in use. More importantly, you must maintain the proper disinfectant residual in the water at all times, as well as keep the acid/alkaline balance (pH) between 7.2 and 7.8. Consequently, a regular maintenance program is an absolute must if you intend to run an energy-efficient pool. Your pump and filter will have to work overtime—and therefore draw more energy—if the filter, the skimmer, and the strainer baskets are clogged with debris. So keep them clean. When you clean the filter, be very careful to follow the manufacturer's instructions; a properly cleaned filter reduces the time you need to circulate your pool water and prevents the pump from becoming overloaded and drawing more electricity.

At the same time, reconsider how often you backwash your filter. Remember that you are spilling gallons and gallons of water away during the backwash process. Without question, the manufacturer's instructions must be followed, but backwashing more than necessary wastes water.

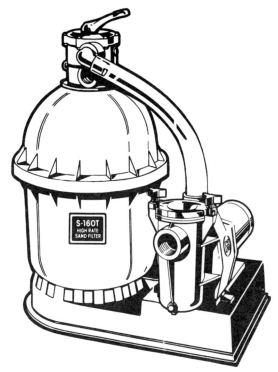

A sand filter.

BACKWASHING A SAND FILTER

Whenever dirt removed from the water clogs a sand filter enough to interrupt the proper flow, the filter should be backwashed.

Most filters have two pressure gauges. One of these reads the pressure at the top of the filter and the other one measures the pressure at the bottom. Generally, when the difference in pressure is between 5 and 7 psi, the filter needs cleaning and should be backwashed. If there are no gauges, sand and gravel filters should be backwashed once a week and/or according to their manufacturer's instructions.

During the process of backwashing a sand filter, the top part of the bed, which consists of graded silica sand, is lifted and scoured. Since the sand is heavier than the debris that has collected on top of it, it remains in the filter tank while the refuse is flushed through the waste line. The backwashing process need only take a few minutes before the waste water turns clear, at which point the filter valves are turned back to their filter position so that the normal filtering process can continue.

The water forced through the filter in a direction opposite to the normal filtering flow is, of course, waste water. It can often be disposed of down a storm drain or into a dry well or two, or a sewer. You can also use it for irrigation, providing the chlorine residue in the pool is low enough so as not to damage the plants or trees you are watering. You cannot, by the way, hook

the backsplash line to a sprinkler or any small diameter line that will restrict its flow, or you will not get the proper backwash action.

Control of the filtered water is a function of the filter underdrain, which is located at the bottom of the sand filter tank. During the filtering operation, the drain collects water passing down through the sand and directs it into the return pool line. But in the backwash process, the underdrain distributes water back up through the sand bed, causing it to be cleaned of its accumulated dirt. If the flow of water through the underdrain is in any way restricted, the backwash action will be insufficient to clean the sand and eventually the filter will stop working. Usually, the underdrain fails because of a buildup of rust or corrosion and calcium deposits from the water. It pays to check the drain from time to time and clean it if necessary.

Another way you can keep your filter operating at peak efficiency is to put a sterilizing compound in the filter every few weeks. The sterilizing chemicals are specially formulated to dissolve body oil, suntan lotions, and grease from the filter bed so that dirt, hair, and other matter are free to be removed during the backwash process. Simply add some of the chemical preparation to the sand bed in the filter before you backwash it and it will act to get your filter sand really clean.

MAINTAINING DIATOMITE FILTERS

The maintenance of diatomite filters is generally simpler than sand filters and while manufacturers usually do not recommend their products be backwashed, the elements must be cleaned regularly to avoid clogging. You may even have to clean the elements more often than you would backwash a sand filter, but the time you put in on both chores is about the same.

However your filter must be cleaned, do it according to the manufacturer's schedule and instructions. In general, when the flow from your filter becomes noticeably lessened, it is time to clean the elements. You can detect this simply by placing your hand over the return port in the pool. If the flow is reduced, it is time to clean the filter elements, or change the cartridge, if your filter is a cartridge type.

It is necessary to launder the filter elements with a household detergent occasionally to get rid of all the body oils and tiny particles of refuse. Otherwise, use a soft brush to clean the filter leaves, removing as little of the diatomaceous earth from the fabric as possible. Even so, it is usually necessary to add a little new earth to the unit after each cleaning.

VALVES

The filter manifold contains the entire group of gate valves serving your filter (there may be a dial selector valve on the manifold instead of a series of valves). Valves, by their design, will last for years without maintenance, but it is still a good idea to inspect them once in a while. Loose packing, particularly in the main drain or vacuum valves, will permit air to enter the filter. If this air is not relieved, it can accumulate at the top of the filter and lower the water level in the filter tank. While filters often have an air release valve or line to prevent air from breaking down the filter media, the drain and vacuum valves ought to be repacked if they are loose.

Dial selector valves sometimes have a lubri-

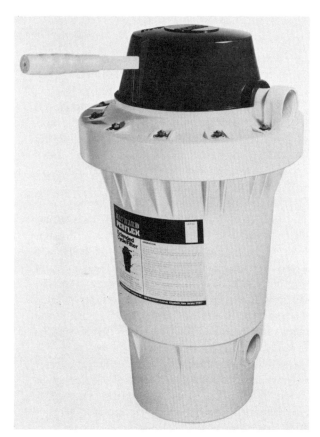

A diatomite earth filter.

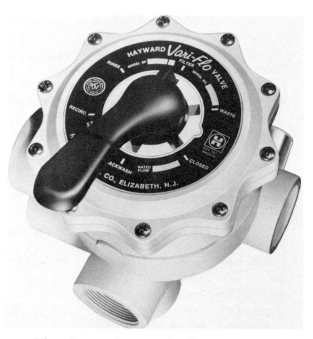

The valves used to control a filter system.

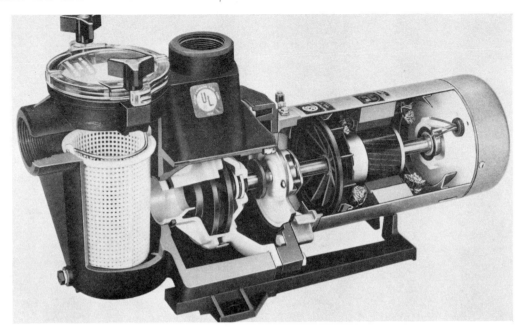

Filter pump and motor.

cating screw that can be given a turn or two to force a self-contained lubricant into the valve to prevent its contact surfaces from binding. Eventually, you will have to replace the lubricant by removing the screw and inserting a replacement grease stick in the hole, then tightening the screw again. Otherwise, consult the valve manufacturer's manual for lubricating instructions.

PUMPS AND MOTORS

Pump motors are electrically powered and demand little or no maintenance. Some require periodic oiling, but most are sealed units that need no lubrication at all. You do have to be careful that all of the electrical connections to the motor are well protected from the weather or any other form of moisture.

The pumps are attached directly to the motor shaft and again the manufacturer's oiling and greasing schedule for all bearings should be followed religiously, and precisely. Do not over-oil either a pump or its motor.

If the pump has a mechanical seal, it is vital that you never run it "dry," that is with insufficient lubricant, or you will burn out the bearings in a matter of minutes. Pumps with a packing gland use water as their lubricant, but these glands can be tightened so much that the shaft

runs dry and will burn out. In lieu of any specific instructions from the manufacturer, allow three or four drops of water to drip out of the packing gland per minute. This type of pump is normally placed in a pit. Be sure the pit has ample drainage and that the drain line is unclogged. If water in the bottom of the pit is allowed to reach the motor, it can short out the electrical contacts and you will be in for a major overhaul or buying a new motor.

When it is time for you to replace your pool pump, its motor, or the filter, have a pow-wow with a reputable pool supplier to decide whether you can install a different-sized unit that would be more energy efficient; at least take a hard look at some of the new, energy-saving pool motors that have been developed in recent years.

PUMP STRAINERS

As water leaves a pool on its way to the filter, it first passes through a strainer which traps most of the hair, lint, leaves, and other large materials before they get into the filter pump and damage it. The strainer is a metal or plastic screen-type basket with an airtight cover that is easily removed, and it should be checked frequently and emptied whenever there is any debris in it. You

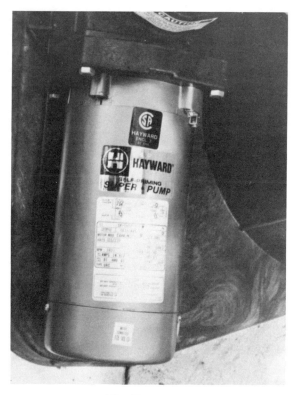

The filter pump.

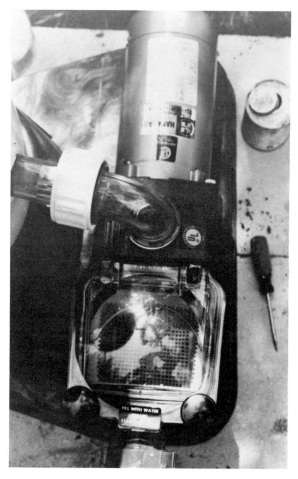

The pump strainer.

can often tell whether the strainer is full just by placing your hand over any of the pool inlets. If you feel little or no suction, the chances are good that the strainer needs cleaning. As a matter of course the strainer should also be emptied whenever you back-flush a sand filter or clean a diatomite filter.

SKIMMERS

Automatic skimmers are supposed to handle half of all the water going from the pool to the filter. But you have to do some work to keep them operating efficiently:

1. Maintain the proper water level in your pool at all times.

2. Be sure the control valve is set to permit a sufficient amount of water to pass through the skimmer.

3. Check the valve on the equalizer line occasionally to be sure it is working properly. Corrosion can cause the valve to leak, permitting water to pass through the equalizer line instead of going over the floating weir. In other words, no

skimming action will take place.

4. Never add any chemicals to the pool through the skimmer, unless you are sure they will not corrode any metal parts in the system.

5. Follow the manufacturer's instructions exactly.

HEATERS

If you believe a pool cover will dramatically reduce the waste of energy, think what happens when you stop using your pool heater so much. Believe it or not, you can make some drastic reductions in pool heating time and not affect your swimming comfort one iota, or even the amount of time you actually spend in the water.

To begin with, consider the temperature of your pool water. Medical authorities insist the most healthful temperature for bathing water is

78° F. Period. For every degree above 78° F., the energy requirement increases by 10 percent. So set the heater thermostat at 78° F. and lock it. Then throw away the key. If you jump in the pool and think the water is too cold, wait awhile; your body will adjust to a 78° F. temperature long before jacking up the heater can possibly raise the temperature of the water as little as even half a degree.

Also consider your swimming season, and be realistic about it. Do you really use your pool every day in December? Or in March for that matter? You could be arbitrary and just lop off two weeks or a month at each end of the season, because NSPI studies have shown that if you predetermine your season, you can save at least 33 percent of all the energy you will use during the entire season.

You should also take a hard look at how long your heater is operating in relation to how much time the pool is actually in use. It might surprise you to discover you are warming up the ol' swimmin' hole for hours every day at great expense when nobody is around to enjoy it.

As your children mature, the patterns of family lifestyle change. When they are adolescents, there is someone in the pool all the time. When they become young adults, family swimming may dwindle to weekends and other special occasions, at which point you can save considerable energy by exerting manual rather than continuous thermostatic control over the water. It requires less energy to heat your swimming pool for a weekend than to keep it at a constant 78° F. temperature all week long.

If you don't have an on-off switch on your heater that can override the thermostat, install one. Or use the thermostat as a switch. On weekends or special occasions, turn the thermostat "on" to 78° F. four hours before you want to swim, and after the party is over switch it to "off," say at 60° F.

Another possibility is to connect your heater to the filtration timer so that it will operate in concert with the filter only during the same hours as the filter is run. You will save considerable energy, particularly if you have calibrated the filter pump to operate around peak utility use times.

Keep trash or leaves from accumulating around the burner draft port; they can cause the burner to burn more fuel than necessary. If you are away from your home for more than two weeks, and at the end of the season, turn the heater off completely, including its pilot light; the heater should be carefully inspected and serviced by a professional before the new season begins.

When you reach the point when you must replace your present heater, carefully compare the thermal efficiency of the various heaters available on the market. Gas- and oil-fired heaters are generally more cost-effective than electric ones. But also consider increasing the size of your heater. A pool needs the same amount of heat no matter what kind of unit provides it. A large heater can supply that heat more quickly, and, therefore, can be used only when you plan to use the pool because it will warm up the water in relatively short order. A heater that is too small not only uses a lot of energy doing its job over a long period of time, but will also allow considerable heat loss during the heat-up period.

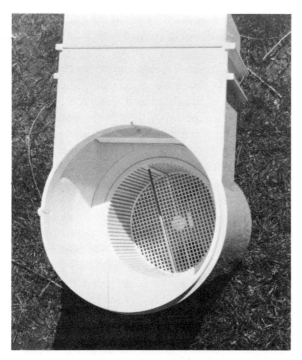

An automatic skimmer.

CLEANING

You can save considerable water by cleaning your pool with a broom instead of a hose. If you have a tile spray, don't use it. Scrubbing tile by

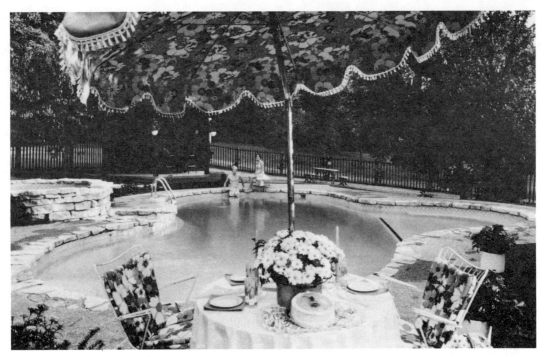

The family's pattern of swimming changes as children grow through their adolescent years and then leave home.

hand is more effective at keeping it shiny anyway.

By applying the same program for your automatic pool cleaner as your filtration system, that is by establishing a minimum cleaning time (about thirty minutes to an hour), you can conserve even more energy, although on unusually dusty days you may have to increase the cleaning time in half-hour increments until the pool is clean. Remember to turn off the pool cleaner whenever the filter pump is not operating.

A pool vacuum differs from the conventional house vacuum only in that it draws water through it instead of air to create suction in the cleaner head. There is also a standard procedure to follow when you vacuum the bottom and sides of your pool, a chore which should be done roughly once a week:

1. Check the vacuum's owner's manual to determine which of the pool valves must be opened or closed during the cleaning operation.

2. Empty the strainer basket and replace it.

3. If it is also time to clean your filter, do it before you do any vacuuming.

4. Close the main suction and skimmer valves, or the main outlet and skimmer line on the filter.

5. Close the air relief valve on the filter.

6. Remove the plug from the vacuum fitting in the pool wall.

7. Attach the hose floats and connect the vacuum hose to the vacuum cleaning head. The floats should be evenly spaced along the hose.

8. Make sure the water level in the pool is well above the vacuum fitting in the pool wall.

9. Attach the cleaner handle to the cleaner head, and submerge the head in the shallow end of the pool. Water will enter the hose; feed the hose into the water as fast as it fills. When the hose is completely full of water (and there is no air in it) it will sink as far as the floats allow it. At that point you can connect the open end of the hose to the vacuum fitting.

10. Turn on the vacuum pump/motor and push the vacuum slowly across the pool floor, working your way toward the deep end.

11. When you are finished vacuuming, empty the strainer basket again and return all of the valves to their filter-operation positions.

CLEANING TIPS

Vacuuming uses electricity, which is an expensive form of energy, and sometimes it may not be necessary to vacuum at all. For example, if you brush down the pool a day or two before you intend to vacuum, matter removed from the walls will settle to the floor of the pool. This may eliminate the necessity of spending time and electricity vacuuming the walls. In fact, if the accumulation of dirt is not appreciable, you may be able just to brush everything into the main drain and let the strainer and filter take care of it.

Remember that when you are brushing down a pool, the main outlet line should be operating, but the skimmer and vacuum lines must be closed so that all available water flow will come only from the deepest part of the pool.

The pool deck should be cleaned frequently, either by hosing or brushing, so that surface dirt does not have an opportunity to be blown into the pool water. It is more energy conserving to sweep the deck every other day than to vacuum your pool once a week.

Don't let any leaves or other large debris that land on the pool surface stay there for very long. When things like leaves become waterlogged and sink to the bottom of the pool, they are difficult to clean up, and they will stain the floor.

CLEANING THE TILE BAND

The 4″ to 6″ tile band around the perimeter of your pool at the water line is not only attractive, but serves to catch hair and body oils, dust, and other minutiae that find their way to the surface of the water before the stuff clogs the skimmer. All of this scum can make your pool look like a dirty bathtub with a ring around it, so you have to clean the tiles once in a while.

The easiest way of cleaning tile is to put pool-tile cleaner, or any good household cleaner, on a sponge or cloth and use a little elbow grease. Tiles are so easy to clean that it should not take more than a few minutes of work.

If a hard white film appears on the tile along the water line, you have a calcium deposit from the water and the water is not properly condi-

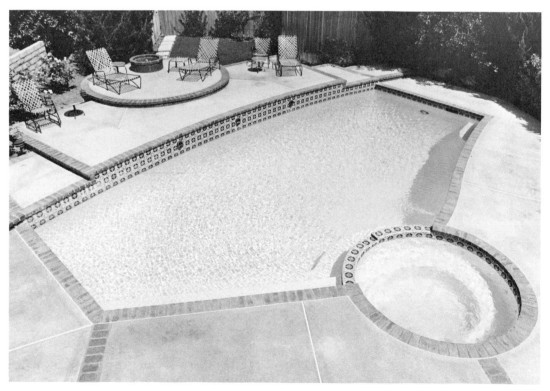

The tile band around the top of your pool is easily wiped clean.

tioned. You are about to have a lot more trouble than just cleaning the tile. The cleaning, however, can be accomplished with a mild solution of one part muriatic acid to six parts water. Don't touch the acid solution with bare hands; it will burn holes in your skin. Wear rubber gloves to wipe the acid solution over the white streaks.

DIVING BOARDS

It is said that a diving board can cause more trouble than the whole rest of a pool. If that is true, it is not because of the board itself, but because it has been improperly installed and maintained. There are five immutable rules to observe with any diving board, no matter what its construction.

1. When the unit is being installed, be certain the board is perfectly aligned with its fulcrum. If it is out of alignment, it will twist and be weakened.

2. Be sure that all of the anchors holding the board in place are firmly fixed to the deck and have no movement whatsoever.

3. When the board is bolted to its anchors, tighten the bolt nuts until the board is held firmly in place, but not with excessive pressure. By overtightening the bolts you can cause a crushing effect that will weaken the board.

4. No horseplay. There shouldn't be any fooling around anywhere near a pool in general, and certainly not on the diving board. Jumps and dives should be taken only from the front of the board. No more than one person should be on the board at one time. The dives people take from a residential pool board should be kept simple. If you have somebody in your family who wants to try out for the Olympics, buy a pool and diving equipment designed for that kind of activity.

5. Make certain that the surface of the board is nonslip and always in perfect repair.

WINTERIZING YOUR POOL

You could carefully maintain and care for your pool all through the swimming season, then walk away from it for a couple of months during the winter and discover that while your back was turned, it did not take care of itself. Come spring, you could discover your nice expensive pool has been severely damaged, or even destroyed. So it is best you perform some off-season maintenance procedures before you close your pool for the winter.

FREEZING

The primary enemy of any pool during the winter is moisture in the ground that freezes, expands, and exerts tremendous pressure against the walls and floor of your pool. Metal pools have been known to buckle as easily as concrete pools crack, to say nothing of what happens to the pipes attending them. A standard winterization procedure is suggested here, but consider each step in terms of your specific pool and climate:

1. At the end of the swimming season, empty the pool.

2. Wash down the walls and floor of the pool and repair any structural cracks or damaged areas. Allow your repairs to dry.

3. In areas where freezing occurs, the pipes have been buried below the frost line. Theoretically, they do not have to be drained, but don't take any chances. Drain all the recirculating and vacuum lines by opening their connections at the lowest point in their runs.

4. Backwash the filter, allowing at least thirty minutes for the operation, and then drain the filter system. Also, empty the filter of all water by opening the drain plugs at the bottom of the tank. If the filter can be removed from its pipe lines, unhook it and store it in a dry place for the winter.

5. Drain the pump and its hair trap (if it is part of the pump) and leave the drain lines open.

6. Disconnect all electrical wires.

7. Store the pump in a dry place for the winter, although actually, only the motor needs to be stored. If you can remove the motor from its pump, the pump can be left outdoors so long as there is no water in it. In any case, grease all of its moving parts and repack the pump shaft packing.

8. Paint the filter system and all exposed metal piping before the bad weather sets in. Wire brush any rust spots, then coat them with red lead primer and a finish coat of metal paint.

9. If you have a removable skimmer, remove it. Built-in skimmers should be drained and filled with rags to absorb moisture. Also cover the

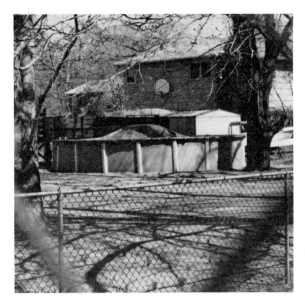

A pool, covered for the winter.

deck grill with a rubber mat or plug so that water cannot enter the skimmer and freeze inside it.

10. Seal the vacuum well with a gasket and plug.

11. Plug the inlet fittings with expandable neoprene or rubber plugs, as well as the bottom outlets and the waste line on the surface skimmer.

12. Plug the main drain.

13. Drain all tanks, pumps, lint catchers, chlorinators, and similar equipment, and remove them from their pipe lines. All of these units should be stored in a dry place for the winter.

14. Remove and store all deck equipment, including all ladders, standards, and the diving board, hoses, and safety ropes.

Inspect all of your equipment carefully for weathering and damage, and make the repairs before you put it away for the winter. If you can't stand the thought of making repairs now, at least make detailed notes about what must be done next spring, before you put the equipment back in service.

15. Fill the pool with water. You could wait until all the leaves have fallen from the trees and then rake them up from the bottom of the pool before you fill it. However, most experts agree it is better to make your repairs and fill the pool immediately.

16. If you expect a thick coating of ice to form on the pool during the winter, you can control excessive expansion of the ice by floating logs or half-filled drums in the water. Anchor such objects in the corners and along the sides of the pool so they will stay in place and not sink or float around, causing damage to the walls of the pool. They can be tied to stakes driven in the ground beyond the edge of the pool.

17. Dump about two gallons of winter algaecide into the water.

18. Stretch some type of nylon, plastic, or canvas cover over the pool. This will prevent leaves and other debris from settling on the water and causing a considerable cleanup chore in the spring (leaves, when they get wet, will stain the finish on most pools). The cover also serves as insulation, and will reduce the effects of the freeze-thaw-freeze cycle as well as protect the paint on the pool. It is also a safety measure so that no one stumbles into the water during the winter. The cover should be secured to stakes driven into the ground beyond the pool walkway.

19. Every two weeks or so during the winter, lift up a corner of the cover and take a look at the water to make sure it is in good condition. If any algae appears, add some more algaecide.

20. In the spring, reinstall all of your equipment and be sure that all of the pieces operate properly. You might consider having a professional pool expert service the filter and heater, just to make sure there is nothing about them that you may have missed. If you decide the interior of your pool needs refurbishing, do it just before you begin the new swimming season.

CHAPTER EIGHT

Water Conditioning

Maintaining the water in your pool is mandatory. Basically, the act of swimming exposes every part of a human being—eyes, ears, nose, all of the skin—to water, and that water must be as pure as you can get it. It must be pure enough to drink at all times or it will cause health problems for swimmers.

While water is one of the basic elements in our lives, it is also so chemically complex that it is rarely perfect in its natural state. It starts out pure enough as it emits from passing clouds, but then it falls through polluted atmospheres and settles into the earth, which imparts a plethora of impurities to it until, by the time it reaches our homes, it contains too much calcium and magnesium, making it "hard," or has too much iron, or too many dissolved solids, or too much algae, or bacteria, or alkalinity, or acidity. When you put it in your pool, the people who swim in it leave traces of body oils, and suntan lotion, and flecks of skin and dirt, and chemicals. The pool very quickly becomes a rather unhealthy body of water unless you execute a continuous and regular program of sterilization for it. That sterilization program consists of adding disinfecting chemicals to the water on a more or less regular basis that depends on the bathing load, the con-

dition of the original water supply, the pool temperature, and the general cleanliness of the pool itself.

CHLORINE—THE FIRST DEFENSE

The standard disinfecting agent recommended by pool and health experts is chlorine, because it has the ability to oxidize organic matter and disease organisms. What oxidation does is literally burn up an organism and kill it.

A portion of the chlorine that you apply to your pool water is immediately consumed in disinfecting the water and is known as the "initial demand" of the water. Whatever active chlorine remains in the water after the "initial demand" is known as the "residual chlorine." It is the residual chlorine content that must be maintained to destroy bacterial and organic matter brought into the pool each day by the climate as well as bathers. Both the initial demand and the residual chlorine are expressed in terms of "parts of available chlorine per million parts of water," or ppm.

In order to manage the water in your swimming pool chemically, you should possess a chemical test kit which, among other things, will allow you to determine the residual chlorine of

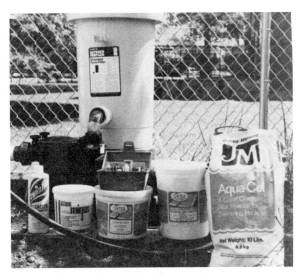

A typical water test kit.

the water. When testing the residual chlorine, a test tube is dipped in different parts of the pool and a few drops of orthotolidine are added to the tube. The water will then take on a color that ranges from clear, which means there is little or no chlorine in the water, to yellow. The deeper the shade of yellow, the more chlorine is present. The shade of yellow is matched with a color scale that comes with the test kit so that you can determine the ppm; the recommended residual chlorine in swimming pool water is between 1.0 and 1.5 ppm. If the water is in this range, it is not only chemically safe, but there is a margin of safety against any further contamination that might enter it.

Chlorine can be purchased as a powder, a liquid, or as granules, and it does not matter how it is added to the pool water, whether by hand or by means of an automatic feeding device known as a chlorinator, as long as the 1.0 to 1.5 ppm level is maintained.

Powdered chlorine (calcium hypochlorite) contains about 70 percent pure chlorine and is sold under several trade names. It has the advantage of not readily deteriorating and being easy to handle and store, and is sold in both powder and tablet form.

Liquid chlorine (sodium hypochlorite) is a solution containing about 16 percent chlorine. As a liquid, sodium hypochlorite is difficult to transport and store for any length of time. If, by the way,

you run out of liquid chlorine, don't turn to a household bleach as a substitute. Products such as Clorox or Purex contain only 5 percent chlorine.

The most recommended form of chlorine to use is a granulated or powdered (dry) stabilized form. "Stabilized" means the chlorine has been mixed with a chemical that resists ultra-violet rays from the sun that can make the chlorine decay rapidly.

MAINTAINING PROPER PPM

In the order of treating pool water with chlorine, if you have just filled your pool and the water has the proper pH (acidity-alkalinity) range, your next step is to superchlorinate the water. By superchlorinating you are dumping between five and ten times the normal amount of chlorine into the pool. Now you have to wait until the residual chlorine is at the recommended 1.0 to 1.5 ppm before you go swimming. From then on, you should test the water daily at several points around the pool and whenever the ppm drops below the 1.0 level, add enough chlorinating concentrate with a built-in stabilizer (to resist the sun) to maintain the 1.0 to 1.5 ppm level. The concentrates can be sprinkled into the pool, or the tablet form can be placed in a floating or in-line chlorine feeder. You will undoubtedly be called upon to superchlorinate your pool several times during the season, depending on the amount of use the pool is getting. The daily dosage of chlorine that is required by the pool may vary with the product you are using. In general, the quantities are:

Pool Capacity In Gallons	Quantity of Powdered Chlorine
Less than 1,000	1 ounce
2,000	3 ounces
3,000	4 ounces
5,000	6 ounces
10,000	8 ounces
15,000	10 ounces
20,000	14 ounces
25,000	18 ounces
50,000	25 ounces

1 ounce = 6 to 8 chlorine tablets
1 ounce = 3 level tablespoons powdered chlorine

If the residual chlorine drops below 1.0 ppm level within a twenty-four-hour period, the original superchlorination was too small, or the pH is too low, causing the chlorine to be used up too quickly. You will have to test the water for its pH level and make the appropriate balancing adjustments. If that fails, the next step would be to superchlorinate again.

DISPENSING CHLORINE

There are several ways of injecting chlorine into your pool. One method is to put twenty-four to thirty-two tablets in a sprinkling can full of water and stir them with a stick until they are dissolved. Remove the head from the can and walk around the pool pouring the solution into the water. You should not mix more than 4 ounces of tablets at a time, so you may have to refill the can a few times until you have put the correct amount of chlorine into your pool. When you reach the bottom of the watering can, you may find a chalky residue. Dump this in the trash, not your pool; all the chlorine has already been spent

from it, and the chalk will only make your water cloudy and then settle on the pool floor.

Another way of dispensing the granules or tablets of chlorine is to put several tablets in dispensing baskets and hang them a few inches below the water surface. At least one basket should be placed on each side of the pool; the tablets will dissolve slowly, providing chlorine to the water for an extended period of time.

You can also equip yourself with an automatic chlorinator that will feed the correct amount of chlorine into the water at the proper time to maintain the ppm level.

Regardless of how you inject chlorine into your pool water, remember that it is a powerful bleaching agent and as such it will cause spots on your clothing. In its full-strength state, it is also not very healthful for human skin, so avoid using the pool for at least a half an hour to an hour after the pool has been treated, depending on the size of the dose you have applied. Actually, because of the effect of chlorine on bathers and the effect of direct sunlight on the chemicals, it is best to do your chlorinating early in the morning or during evening hours.

pH—THE SECOND DEFENSE

The second most important factor in proper water management is the control of its acid/alkaline balance, or potential Hydrogen (pH). The symbol pH represents an arbitrary numerical scale from 0 to 14 that is used to indicate the acidity-alkalinity balance of water. A pH of 7.0 is dead neutral. All values from 7.0 down to 0 indicate too much acid. It has been established that the pH of water should range between 7.2 and 7.8 for the ideal bather comfort level. In fact, when you jump in a pool and the water irritates your eyes and nose, it is not because of too much chlorine, but because the water is too acidic.

Aside from the bathers' comfort there are a number of other reasons for maintaining the proper pH in your pool water. If the water becomes even slightly acidic, it will attack the pool surfaces, causing abrading and roughness; if the pool is made of cement, it will eat away the surface and expose the sand aggregate underneath. Ignore an unbalanced pH condition for only a few days and you are in for a complete resurfacing job on your pool. Overly acid water will also

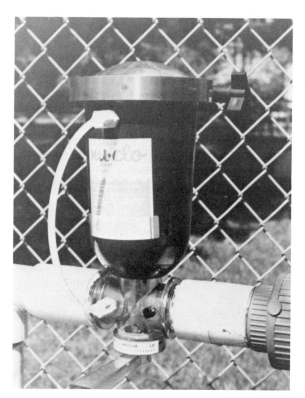

An automatic chlorinator.

damage your filter and piping, and dissolve any galvanizing and other protective coatings on metal parts. And if the acid/alkaline unbalance reaches a level of 8.0 or more on the pH scale, the water will calcify in the pool heater and leave hard-to-remove calcium deposits on the pool walls and floor.

Moreover, an unbalanced pH in your water will reduce the benefits you get from the algaecides and chlorine you put in the pool. The sterilizing agents you use are the major cause of any change in pH. Chlorine will raise the pH in proportion to how much of it is put in the water, and therefore you may also have to inject a compensating amount of acid. If the pH falls below 7.0, the chlorine will tend to dissipate, which lowers the residual chlorine content in the water, to say nothing of the rather disagreeable odor it imparts to the water.

The only way you can determine the pH of your pool water is to test it with a water test kit. The kits are not expensive and they come with all the scales, measures, and chemicals you need to keep track of both the pH and the chlorine level. With most kits you fill a test tube with pool water and then add a measured amount of reagent, which is usually phenol red. Then you shake the tube to mix the phenol red with the water and watch the water change from a light yellow to red or purple. You can then compare the color of the water with a color scale provided in the kit. Each color is marked with its correct pH degree.

If the water is below 7.2 on the color scale (orange) it has too much acid in it and you will have to add soda ash to it to give it more alkalinity. To do this, place a pound of soda ash for every 5,000 gallons of pool water in two gallons of water to dissolve it, then pour it around the swimming pool. An hour later take another pH test; if the water is still below the 7.2 level, add more soda ash and continue adding it until you reach the proper chemical balance.

If the pH is too alkaline, an acid such as sodium bisulphate or muriatic acid is added to the pool water. The sodium bisulphate is a powder and muriatic acid comes in liquid form. Both chemicals can cause skin irritation, so when working with them wear rubber gloves. The sodium bisulphate is mixed with a pail of water at a ratio of 1 pint for every 5,000 gallons of pool water. If your initial dosage fails to bring the pH

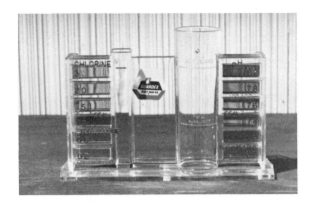

The pH scale on a water test kit.

level down to the 7.2 to 7.8 range, add more chemical at two-hour intervals until it does.

Alkalinity helps to keep the pH in proper range and the pool water balanced, so it should be watched carefully and tested at least once a week. Bathers can enter the pool immediately after a dosage of sodium bisulphate, muriatic acid, or soda ash is applied and in fact their movement will help the chemicals react more quickly. The water should have a proper pH balance before any chlorine or algaecides are added to it so their chemical action is not impaired.

THE AGONIES OF ALGAE

Algae is a plant growth nourished by sunlight and heat that can appear in both a free-floating or a clinging form. It turns the water green, or cloudy, causes spots on the pool walls, and creates slippery surfaces all over the place. Algae thrive in water that has a high pH and if you don't stop it the moment you see it, it can cover your whole pool in a matter of hours and begin fostering bacteria. If it gets really out of hand, the pool must be drained and the walls and floor scrubbed with full-strength chlorine.

If you keep your pool at the recommended pH level and properly chlorinated at all times, the chances of algae appearing are reduced, but not eliminated. But if you skip a day or two of chlorination, or there is a heavy bathing load during very hot weather, the algae may appear anyway. At which point, superchlorinate the water by adding between five and ten times the normal dosage of chlorine and the pool may regain its clarity in less than an hour. Immediately brush any spots of loose algae from the walls and floor and vacuum the pool, then test the water for residual chlorine, and make sure it is between 1.0 and 1.5 ppm.

If you are afraid that algae may occur, you might supplement your normal chlorine treatments by adding a pint of copper sulphate once a week, or better still, use one of the special algaecides available at pool suppliers. The algaecide should be applied according to its manufacturer's instructions, which generally will call for no more than once or twice a week unless the weather is really hot and the sunlight unusually bright. Most algaecides are liquids that are poured into the pool and distributed through the water by the normal agitation of bathers. But remember, no algaecide is a replacement for chlorine, only a supplement.

OTHER WATER TROUBLES

The water in your pool demands a constant vigil or it will abruptly stop being clear and sanitary. Some of the problems that can arise and ways to solve them are:

CLOUDY WATER

The water can turn cloudy because of algae, water hardness, frequent backwashing, an insufficient filter, precipitating calcium compounds, improper pH, total alkalinity, or dissolved solids. Whatever the reason for the cloudiness, there are several steps you can take to retrieve your water clarity.

1. Be sure you are maintaining a 1.0 to 1.5 ppm residual chlorine level.
2. Be sure the pH is in the 7.2 to 7.8 range at all times.
3. Run your filter continuously until the water is clear again.
4. Inspect the filtration system and be sure it is functioning perfectly.

DISCOLORED POOL FINISH (Scale)

This could come from calcium deposits or algae growth.

1. Treat the water with an algaecide.
2. If the problem is calcium deposits you may have to install a water softener on the pool filter line. But there may be some dissolved solids in

the water as well, which could make removal of the discoloration tricky. It is best to consult a local pool expert about what the deposits contain and how to remove them. He should be able to recommend procedures and products to eliminate the problem.

FOAMING

If your water develops what looks like soap bubbles on its surface, there is too much algae or organic debris in it.

1. Follow the instructions for use on the algaecide package.
2. Discard as much water as is necessary.
3. Superchlorinate.
4. Maintain the proper pH and residual chlorine.

TOO MUCH IRON

Iron, manganese, and/or metallic salts are present in the water of many locales around the country. They do not make the water undrinkable, but they can give your pool water an unsavory reddish hue, and eventually stain the pool interior. One solution is to install an iron filter in your pool support system. If that is unfeasible, try this:

1. Completely fill the pool and turn on the filter system.
2. Fill a burlap bag with alum and tie it to a stick; then dunk the bag in the pool vigorously until most of the alum has dissolved.
3. Superchlorinate the pool.
4. Run the filter continuously and backwash it every time the pressure differential reaches 5 to 7 psi. You may have to do this every couple of hours because of the heavy load on the filter.
5. Check the pH every two hours. If the pH falls below 7.0, start adding soda ash in small quantities until the pH is over 7.2.
6. When the water is clear, vacuum the sides and floor thoroughly.

DISSOLVED SOLIDS

Any water supply that has an excess of dissolved solids will constantly leave some of them on the walls of the pool, particularly if they are the calcium salts found in hard water. The calcium will leave white streaks on the pool surfaces and clog the heater pipes and perhaps even the filter.

The best solution is usually to add regularly a sequestering agent such as sodium hexametaphosphate or ethylenediaminetetraacetic acid (EDTA). These will help, but there will still be a buildup of dissolved solids, so you will have to empty the pool, scour it, then refill it at least once every year.

WATER TEST KITS

There are dozens of water test kits available today, representing a range of test capabilities as well as price. Unless your area has unusual water problems, the kit you buy need only be able to measure residual chlorine and the degree of pH. No matter what type or quality kit you own, to get the best test results remember to follow these basic points:

1. Always follow the kit manufacturer's procedures exactly when making each test.

2. Rinse your hands briskly in the pool before handling any of the reagents that come with the kit. The reagents are very sensitive and perspiration or dirt on your hands might inadvertently be introduced into the test tube, resulting in an incorrect reading.

3. Wash the test tube carefully and thoroughly after each use. Any residue left in the tube could affect the next reading you take from the tube.

4. Some or all of the chemicals used with a water kit cannot be relied on from one year to another. It is best to purchase a new supply of reagents at the beginning of each swimming season and throw out their remains when you close your pool for the winter.

5. The color standards that are a part of the kits rely on specific hues produced by the kit manufacturer's chemicals. When replacing any of the chemicals, try to get them from the same company that made the kit.

6. Always store your water test kit in a dry, warm place. The liquids in the kit can be harmed by both direct sunlight and freezing temperatures.

CHAPTER NINE

Trouble-Shooting Pools

A constant maintenance program will keep the water in your pool sanitary and your equipment in good working order. But even the best-cared-for pools can develop troubles that must be located and repaired. Here are the most common pool ailments and what to do about them.

FILTERS

The biggest problems that arise with filters are caused by air leaks in the filtration system. The first indication of such leaks on the suction side of the pump may be excessive air bubbles entering the pool from the return fitting, or air blowing back through the main drain or surface skimmer when the filter is turned off, or pressure gauges vibrating or not registering at all. If the leakage is on the discharge side of the pump, it will announce itself by a bubbling sound in the filter tank every time the filter is turned off:

FILTER TROUBLE-SHOOTING CHARTS

PROBLEM: AIR LEAK IN FILTER SYSTEM

CAUSE	SOLUTION
Water too low	Raise water level
Pump packing loose	Tighten mechanical seals; repack pump
Valve packing loose	Repack valves
Pump strainer lid loose	Tighten lid
Leak in suction pipe or fittings	Repair or replace pipe and fittings

PROBLEM: PRESSURE DROPS; SUCTION DECREASES

CAUSE	SOLUTION
Clogged suction lines	Flush out lines
Clogged pump	Dismantle and clean pump

PROBLEM: FILTER CIRCULATES BUT DOES NOT FILTER WATER

CAUSE	SOLUTION
Tipped filter tank	Level tank
Channeled filter bed of filter media caked	Backwash filter; if a channel remains, empty and refill filter tank

POOL PUMP TROUBLE-SHOOTING CHARTS

PROBLEM: LITTLE OR NO WATER DELIVERED

CAUSE	SOLUTION
No prime	Fill pump and suction completely with water
Speed too low	Check whether motor is receiving full voltage or has an open phase
Discharge head too high	Check pipe friction losses; larger piping may correct condition; are valves wide open?
Suction lift too high	If no obstruction at inlet, check for pipe friction losses; if static lift too high, water may need to be raised or pump lowered
Impeller plugged	Remove pump casing and clean impeller
Air leaks in suction piping	Little water delivered; test flanges for leakage with flame or match; seal any leaks
Air in stuffing box	Adjust gland to produce proper tightness or repack; clean water seal piping; center lantern ring at water seal piping
Not enough positive suction head for hot water	Check with pump manufacturer
Defective wearing rings	Replace if worn excessively
Defective impeller	Replace if damaged or blades eroded
Defective packing	Replace packing, and sleeves, if worn
Foot valve too small or partially obstructed	Area through ports of valve should be at least as large as area of suction pipe—preferably 1½ times; if strainer is used, net clear area should be three or four times area of suction pipe
Suction inlet not immersed deep enough	If inlet cannot be lowered—or if swirling eddies through which air is sucked persist when it is lowered—chain a board to suction pipe; it will be drawn into eddies, smothering the vortex.

PROBLEM: PUMP STOPS OCCASIONALLY

CAUSE	SOLUTION
Incomplete priming	Air-tighten pump, piping, and valves
Suction lift too high	Check for obstruction at inlet, and pipe friction losses; if static lift too high, water to be pumped must be raised or pump lowered
Air leaks in suction piping	Seal all leaks; adjust gland or add new
Air leaks in stuffing box	packing; water seal piping may be plugged and need cleaning; lantern ring may be displaced—center at water seal piping
Air in water	Overrate pump to provide adequate pressure despite condition; watch for bubble formation

PROBLEM: PUMP DRAWS TOO MUCH POWER

CAUSE	SOLUTION
Head lower than rating, pumps too much water	Turn down impeller's outside diameter in amount advised by your pump manufacturer
Stuffing boxes too tight	Release gland pressure or replace packing
Casing distorted	Check alignment; examine pump for friction between impeller and casing, worn wearing rings; replace damaged parts
Misalignment	Realign pump and motor

PROBLEM: NOT ENOUGH PRESSURE

CAUSE	SOLUTION
Speed too low	Check whether motor is directly across the line and receiving full voltage; or frequency may be too low, motor may have an open phase; correct
Air in water	Try to overrate pump to provide adequate pressure despite condition; watch for bubble formation
Too small impeller diameter	Check with your pump manufacturer to see if a larger impeller can be used; otherwise, cut pipe losses, or increase speed—or both, as needed

HEATER TROUBLE-SHOOTING CHARTS

PROBLEM: FLAMES COMING FROM SIDES OF HEATER

CAUSE	SOLUTION
Too much water flowing through heater	Adjust water flow according to instructions
Lack of adequate air	Provide adequate air supply to heater
Improper venting	Provide proper venting of heater

Burner shutters adjusted improperly	Adjust burner shutters properly
Burner clogged with corrosion	Remove and clean burners; adjust water flow properly
Thermometer missing, broken, or incorrectly installed	Install thermometer
Time clock out of adjustment	Adjust time clock properly
Gas burning at orifice (flashback)	Check nameplate for correct gas; consult factory for corrective measures

PROBLEM: HEATER DOES NOT HEAT WATER PROPERLY

CAUSE	SOLUTION
Time clock incorrectly set; filter is off too much of the time	Reset clock to let heater operate continuously
Filter dirty	Clean filter frequently
Thermostat out of adjustment or defective	Test thermostat—recalibrate or replace if necessary
Pressure switch defective	Adjust pressure switch or replace
Gas line too small	Have pool builder or gas company recommend proper pipe size
Heater too small	Replace with larger unit

PROBLEM: SCALE ON HEATER TUBES

CAUSE	SOLUTION
Heater improperly installed	Install according to instructions
Thermometer missing, broken, or incorrectly installed	Install thermometer
Heater stays "on" when filter flow diminishes	Adjust or replace pressure switch

PROBLEM: HEATER DOES NOT TURN ON

CAUSE	SOLUTION
Pool filter or pump strainer clogged or dirty	Clean filter and strainer
Pump air-locked, clogged, inoperative	Clean or repair pump
Main drain and/or skimmer valves closed	Set normal valve settings for skimmer and main drain
Water flow through heater out of adjustment	Adjust water flow through heater
Plugged tee-strainer	Remove plug and clean tee-strainer
Pilot out	Clean orifice; relight pilot
Pilot generator defective	Check output of pilot generator with millivolt meter; replace if necessary

Broken wiring, loose or corroded connections	Inspect for breaks, clean terminals; trace out circuit
Controls out of adjustment or calibration, or defective	Adjust controls; replace if necessary
Electric gas valve inoperative	Replace electric gas valve if necessary
Gas shut off	Open gas valve

REPAINTING

It is generally conceded that the interior finish of a pool is the most important part of its construction and there are four types of interior finishes that have proven themselves over the years to be the most durable. The most common finish is paint, then there are plastered finishes applied with a trowel, built-in plastic liners and fiberglass, and finally tile. Tile has become so expensive it is now almost a prohibitive material, but paint, plaster, and plastic are all within the means of most pool owners.

TYPES OF POOL PAINT

The three paint types recommended for covering pool interiors are cement-based, which comes as a powder that must be mixed with water, chlorinated rubber-based paint, and the type made of plastic resins. Standard oil-based paints and enamels are unable to resist the softening effects of water so they are not deemed as practical. Among the three preferred paint types, you will find a full range of colors. The rubber- or vinyl-based types can be applied with a brush, roller, or spray gun, and both are judged to be more durable than the cement-based paints.

PREPARING FOR PAINTING

The most important step you take during the process of painting a pool is preparation of the surfaces to be painted. All pool paints depend on a rough surface for their adhesion. If your pool is a brand-new one, a wood-float or a troweled finish etched with acid provides an ideal painting surface. If you are renovating an old pool, sandblasting will produce the appropriate surface texture.

To prepare either a new or an old pool surface for repainting, first wash it thoroughly, removing every trace of scum, body oil, dirt, and grease. You can do your pool cleaning with any household detergent but 1½ ounces of trisodium phosphate (TSP) mixed in a gallon of water together with 1½ ounces of soap chips will do a very credible job and doesn't cost very much. When you are done scrubbing, hose off all of the surfaces and allow them to dry thoroughly.

If you have areas where the old paint is flaked or peeling, buff them with a power sander, or if the work is extensive, rent a sand blaster. Chemical paint removers not only do not work terribly well on concrete, but they leave a waxy residue that even TSP will have a hard time removing.

CRACKS AND SPALLING

A concrete pool may develop cracks more readily during its first year of existence than at any other time because the pool is busy settling into its hole in the ground. If the cracks are hairline, that is, minute surface fissures that do not go deep enough to permit water to seep through them or appreciably disturb the looks of the pool, they will be more or less hidden by a good coat of paint.

When the cracks are large enough to ruin the looks of the pool, or if they are deep enough to let pool water out or ground water in, they must be filled. One way of determining whether a crack goes all the way through the concrete is to hold a face tissue over it. If the tissue is drawn into the crack, you have a leak.

To fill large cracks, enlarge them with a cold chisel, undercutting the edges of the cut so that the old concrete overhangs the edges of the area to form a lock that will hold your patching cement in place. Next clean the area with a wire brush, removing all dirt and loose concrete; then wet the entire area to be patched.

Mix a mortar made of hydraulic cement and force it into the damaged area; then level it off with the surrounding surface. Depending on the mortar you use and its manufacturer's instructions, you should keep the patch wet for anywhere from two hours to three days, until it has completely cured and hardened.

Spalling is really the pitting and roughing of a concrete surface and is caused by the weather and water wearing away at an unprotected portion of the pool surface. The roughness is usually deep enough to require resurfacing with a good patching concrete designed to adhere to old concrete. The patching cement is troweled over the damaged area and provides a smooth-textured finish. First clean the area with a wire brush and if any of the pits are more than a quarter of an inch deep, apply the patching cement in two thin coats, rather than one thick one. Patching cement is available in both mixed and unmixed forms and can be applied with either a trowel or a brush.

ETCHING

Assuming you have a concrete pool that has been cleaned, bared, and properly patched, it is not rough enough for the paint to adhere to properly. So the surfaces must be etched, and the simplest way of doing this is with muriatic acid. One part acid is mixed with ten parts water. This solution is then poured on the concrete and scrubbed with a long-handled brush (long-handled so that you aren't splattered). Allow the acid to effervesce for a time; then flush it off the surfaces with a hose and scrub the concrete to remove all remaining debris.

A warning about muriatic acid: It is dangerous. Always wear rubber gloves and work as far away from it as you can get with long-handled tools. When mixing muriatic acid, always pour the acid into the water, never splash water into the acid.

TEST PAINT

If you are painting over any unknown surfaces, that is, going over old paint, you need to know if the new paint will adhere properly. So apply new paint to several places on the old paint and give it at least two hours to dry. Then examine the new paint for cracking, wrinkling, bleeding, or blistering. If you find any such signs, change

paints or sandblast the old material off the pool surfaces. If there is no change in the texture of the new paint, you can assume the two materials are compatible. But don't continue with your painting yet. Wait twenty-four hours and then scratch the test spots with your fingernail or a light tool. If you cannot separate the two paints easily, you will probably get a satisfactory paint job.

PAINTING MASONRY

Whatever paint you put on a pool, apply it the way the instructions on the container tell you to apply it. Beyond what the manufacturer tells you, here are some other hints to bear in mind:

1. Be sure the paint is thoroughly mixed. Even if it was done on a machine at the paint store, still stir it a little and "box" it, that is, pour it from one can to another and back. There should be no residue left in the cans as you empty them.

2. Don't thin a pool paint any more than you absolutely have to to apply it easily. If you are using a brush or roller, it should need little or no thinning; if you are spraying, use only as much of the manufacturer's recommended thinner as is necessary to make it sprayable. You are painting your pool to give it a protective coating; don't cheat yourself (and the pool) by "stretching" the paint until all you have on the pool surfaces is a touch of color.

3. Pool paint sets quickly. Nevertheless, wait for the first coat to dry overnight before applying the second coat. Also wait the full recommended time (usually a week or so) after the final coat is on before you fill the pool with water.

4. Paint in the shade if at all possible.

PAINTING METAL POOLS

Steel pools absolutely must have all of their surfaces protected by paint or they will develop rust spots, a process which is hastened by any chlorine you are putting in the water. Even aluminum pools require painting and in both instances the metals must be primed with a rust-inhibiting primer before the finish coat is applied. Allow a day or two for the primer to dry.

If you find rusted areas on any metal surface, they should be removed with a power sander (and coarse paper) or a wire brush. Spot prime the buffed areas with the appropriate metal

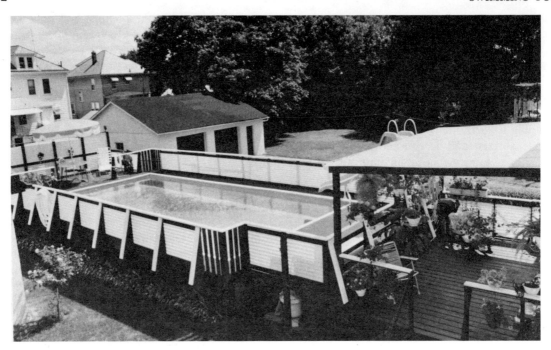

Metal, both steel and aluminum, requires some painting from time to time.

primer and allow twenty-four to forty-eight hours before priming the entire pool. If the rust is exceptionally deep or extensive, consider sandblasting.

The procedure for repainting metal pools is this:

1. Remove all blistering, peeling, or flaking paint, as well as all rust, by scraping with a wire brush or coarse sandpaper or sandblasting.

2. Clean every surface with a detergent to remove all grime, grease, and dirt.

3. Prime all bare metal spots and wait one to two days.

4. Prime all metal surfaces with a rust-inhibiting primer, and allow a day or two for the paint to dry.

5. Apply two coats of finish paint, allowing the proper amount of drying time between each coat, as stated by the paint manufacturer.

NONSKID MATERIALS

Decking, ladders, steps, and particularly diving boards must be covered with a decking material that is nonskid no matter whether it is wet or

dry. It should be immune to chlorine, detergents, and other pool chemicals. It should be cool to walk on, which means it must be capable of dissipating the sun's heat, no matter whether it is applied to wood or metal or masonry.

Some nonskid materials are applied with a brush, others with a trowel. When using the brush-on type, a clear neutralizer is normally applied first to establish a neutral base for the nonskid material. When the base coat has dried the nonskid coating is brushed on. Don't be surprised by it; nonskid materials have lousy flow characteristics so you have to use short, full brush strokes.

With the trowel-on type of nonskid material, you can normally trowel a single coat about 1/32″ thick. If you want a thicker coating than that, permit the first coat to dry and then apply a second coat. Don't try to get it all on with one thick application.

AVOIDING PROBLEMS WITH PAINT

There are a few general rules to bear in mind if you want to avoid problems with the paint you apply to your pool.

1. Avoid "all-in-one" types of paint. They are not as reliable as single-purpose water-resistant paints.

2. If you are constructing a new pool, be certain the drainage system under and around it is good, and that the exterior walls behind the pool are coated with bituminous paint before they are backfilled. This will inhibit ground water from pushing its way through the concrete to dislodge your interior paint.

3. Be certain all surfaces to be painted are clean and dry. The paint cannot adhere to bits of algae, body oil, grit, or anything else.

4. Do not paint any damp surfaces or moisture will be trapped behind the paint and cause it to peel. Allow the concrete to dry properly before painting and don't paint while morning dew or evening moisture is on the surfaces of the pool.

5. The best way to paint is to follow the sun around your pool, always working in the shade. The ideal painting temperatures are between 60° F. and 80° F.

6. Let your fresh paint dry completely before you fill the pool with water.

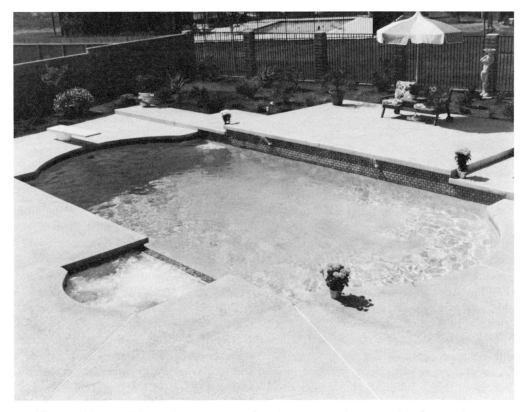

All nonskid materials applied to any surface in or around your swimming pool must remain nonskid no matter what material they are applied to, and what the weather may happen to be.

CHAPTER TEN

Hot Tubs and Spas

Hot tubs and spas are all generally 4′ deep and 4′ to 5′ in diameter. They are distinguished from the everyday variety of tub by their plumbing as well as their size, and they are never used in exactly the same manner as your everyday household bathtub. You fill a normal tub with hot water and then sit in it up to your ears in lather until the water turns lukewarm. Then you pull a plug and all of the water and soap residue is sucked down a drain and disappears into a sewer system. But hot tubs and spas are attended by a plumbing system that includes a filter as well as a pump and a heater. Their design is specifically contrived to recirculate the water through the filter to keep it clean, and to be constantly reheated by the heater to keep it hot for as long as you wish to remain in the tub. Moreover, the process of cleaning and heating the water is helped by the circulating pump, which continuously moves the water, which in turn provides a therapeutic benefit as you are soaking. It is the movement of 100° F. water that has a unique ability to relax taut muscles and wash away the tensions of an overwrought psyche.

Another difference between hot tubs and regular bathtubs is that you cannot use any soap in a hot tub or a spa for the simple reason that you are reusing the water and the filter placed in the circulating system cannot get rid of any detergent residue.

Both hot tubs and spas are traditionally installed outdoors, as part of a patio or deck, perhaps beside a swimming pool, or nestled in a secluded part of the garden, which makes their use more of a seasonal activity than standard tubs. They can, however, be placed indoors with the advantage of more privacy, better control over their environment, and therefore, year-round use. Not everybody thinks of putting on a bathing suit when he or she decides to soak in a hot tub or spa, and sometimes a garden or other outdoor setting cannot afford the seclusion required for soaking in the altogether.

The essential difference between hot tubs and spas is the material used to build them. Hot tubs are normally round, have vertical sides, and are made of unstained redwood, although you can find hot tubs that are oval, rectangular, or square with angled sides made of oak, cypress, or some other durable hardwood. Spas today are usually made of fiberglass molded into a single unit with an inside liner constructed of some hard, polished material, but they can also be metal or concrete. The shape, color, and size of a spa can

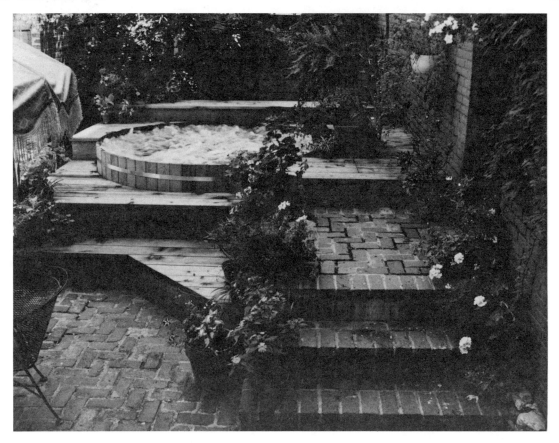

Hot tubs are always made of wood, usually redwood, cedar, or oak.

be just about anything its constructor wants it to be.

For the most part, everything else about spas and hot tubs is identical. They both can be installed indoors or outdoors; they both contain water that health authorities recommend should be maintained at temperatures ranging between 100° F. and 104° F. They both cost less than a swimming pool and require the same basic support equipment. Because they are smaller than pools, tubs and spas can be situated in less space, use less water, less heat, and require less maintenance. Furthermore, they provide a form of physical therapy and relaxation that is at least as old as the Holy Roman Empire and probably even older than that.

A SHORT HISTORY

The ancient Romans, the Egyptians, Greeks, Turks, and Japanese all had some form of com-

munal hot bathing. The Romans may have overdone it a bit with their huge heated public baths that could hold thousands of men, women, and children at a time, all soaking, relaxing, and energetically socializing with their friends. At the other end of the spectrum, the Japanese maintain a centuries-old tradition of family bathing in free-standing wooden vats known as *ofuros*. But only the family and honored guests get into the family tub, not the whole neighborhood.

During the intervening years between the ancient cultures and modern society, the Europeans have soaked in hot tubs and at resort spas that offered hot mineral waters. The tradition of soothing tension and relaxing the mind in steaming hot water was carried to the Americas during colonial times and quickly produced such noted spas as Saratoga Springs, Warm Springs, and Calistoga. These were proliferated by the rich and the socially elite, and longed for by the poor until the late 1960s when a bunch of bohemians living in

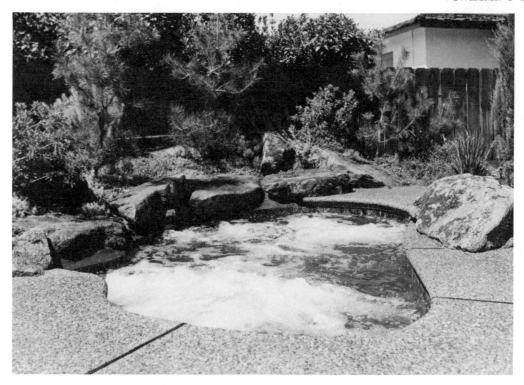

Hot tubs and spas are normally installed outdoors.

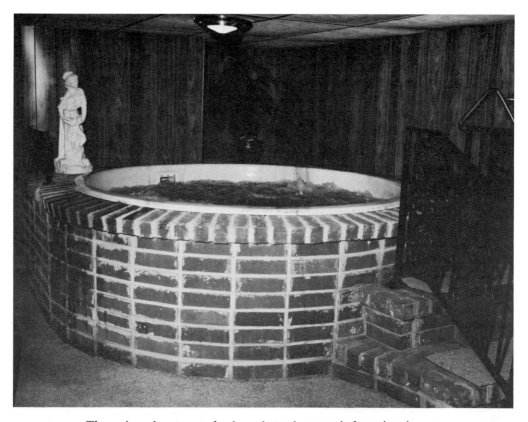

The major advantage to having a hot tub or spa indoors is privacy.

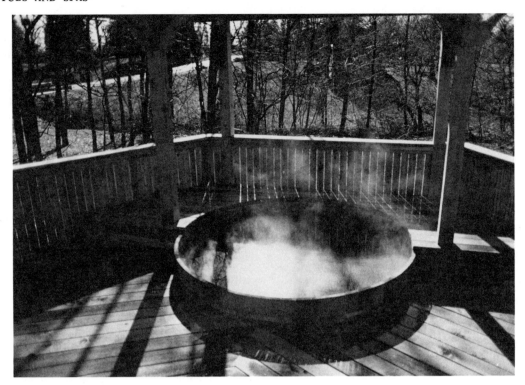

Hot tubs are almost always round or oval.

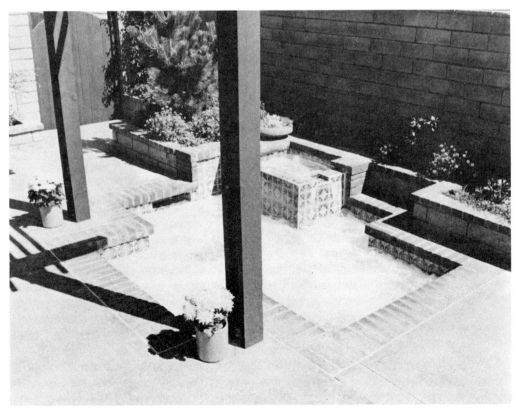

Spas are produced in practically every shape imaginable.

Santa Barbara decided to combine the pure fun of socializing with their neighbors (à la the Romans) with relaxing in their own back yards (à la the Japanese).

The Santa Barbarans scoured the hills of California collecting old wine vats, water tanks, heaters, and pipes, and began to create some pretty weird and wonderful hot tub systems that not only worked, but spawned a whole industry of hot tub and spa companies. Today, the tub systems have been refined, packaged, and merchandised all over the United States, although nothing says you can't go about the business of building your own hot tub, probably at considerably less cost than the going price of around $3,000 installed.

HOT TUB OR SPA?

Your choice between a hot tub or spa is likely to be determined by aesthetics, cost, and available space. The tubs cost less, and if their rustic appearance fits into your landscape or house décor you will most likely select a tub. If the landscaping around your house imposes some limitations, or if the house is decorated in such a way that a polished, sculptured spa is more suitable, then obviously that will be your choice. Unless, of course, the difference in cost places a restriction on your budget.

TUB TYPES

Hot tubs tend to be made of wood and installed above ground level, which gives them the advantage of lower installation costs and a portability that spas normally do not offer. Modern-day hot tubs are made by coopering companies that are likely to be manufacturing wine casks and olive oil kegs as a primary source of revenue. The tubs can be round or oval with their staves held in place by metal hoops. When they are installed, they rest on concrete piers or plates, and the first time you fill the tub it will leak between its staves for a couple of days until the wood swells enough to make the unit watertight. Old wooden barrels, wine vats, and hot tubs are never made with nails or any other fastener to hold the staves together.

The size of a hot tub can vary considerably from 3½′ to 12′ or more in diameter. On an average they are between 5′ and 6′ in diameter and 4′ deep. The depth can vary, but hot tubs are neither swimming pools nor bathtubs so only a specially ordered one would have more or less depth than the norm of 2½′ to 5′. A standard 4′ by 5′ tub can hold 500 gallons of water, and when filled with bathers will weigh between 3½ and 4 tons.

TUB WOODS

The preferred wood used to make hot tubs is vertical-grain all-heart redwood (primarily because redwood has a natural resistance to water); if maintained properly it will last for fifteen years or more.

But there are other woods just as durable and in places where they are available at a reasonable cost, they are just as good. Teak, for example, is about as tough a wood as you can get. But you have to get it on the other side of the world, so it is expensive by the time it reaches America. If you are willing to pay the price, a teak hot tub will last for decades without decay, and offers the plus that it has a natural oily smoothness.

Oak is often used in tubs because it is tough, although it is not resistant to decay and must be carefully and constantly maintained. Then again, people have used oak to build ships for centuries.

Cedar is very close to redwood although it resists chemical damage better and decay not quite as well, which means it may not last quite as long as fifteen years.

All of the woods used in hot tubs should be kiln-dried as opposed to air-dried. Kiln-dried wood tends to absorb moisture more evenly, preventing it from warping or buckling as time and the weather attack it. Whatever wood you select, use the heart wood. Although it is rarer (heart wood is the very center of the tree and like everything else on this planet, trees only have one heart), it is likely to be strongest without any weak spots that water can eventually seep through.

The price of every hot tub is based on the cost of its materials. If you live in California where both cedar and redwood are abundant, an average tub will cost less than if it is manufactured in New Jersey. On the other hand, oak costs twice as much in California as redwood, but in Kentucky, where there are whole forests of oak to

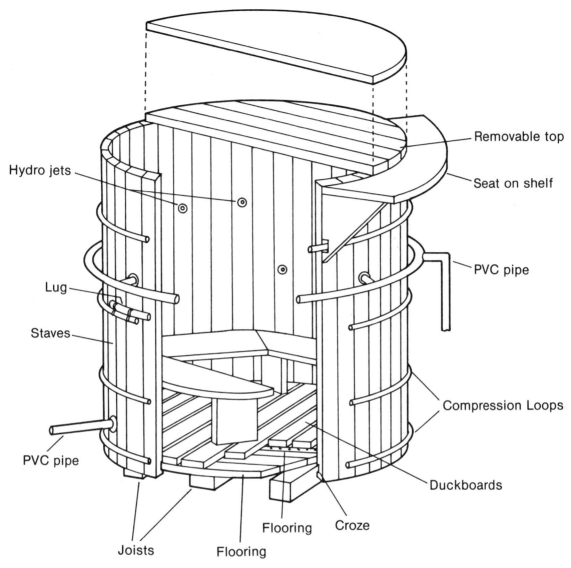

Removable top

Seat on shelf

Hydro jets

PVC pipe

Lug

Staves

Compression Loops

PVC pipe

Duckboards

Croze

Joists

Flooring

Flooring

Anatomy of a wooden hot tub.

pick from, an oak tub is priced about the same as a cedar tub in California.

Roughly, the price of an average-sized wooden hot tub is between $1,000 and $1,500. They are sold, by the way, at a rate of about 40,000 a year in all parts of the United States. But the cost of the vat itself is only half the final expense of purchasing and installing a hot tub. With it, you must have a pump or two (at $100 plus per pump), a filter, a heater, some plumbing, and perhaps an air blower, so your final tab for buying and installing an average hot tub is between $2,000 and $3,000.

There are some ways of cutting the installation cost. If you are really a handyman at heart, you can do some or all of the masonry, plumbing, and electrical work yourself, which eliminates all or part of the expense of hiring a contractor. You can also do your own maintenance, which with hot tubs is a time-consuming (and therefore expensive) proposition. Bear in mind that with the exception of teak, the wood used in the tub is subject to considerable deterioration unless it is cared for on a regular basis.

The one great advantage of hot tubs is that because they are normally installed on concrete piers or plates and stand above the ground, you can take them with you whenever you decide to move.

KINDS OF SPAS

Originally, spas were constructed out of concrete, usually as adjuncts to a swimming pool. In fact, spas are still installed primarily as an addendum to an in-ground swimming pool. The advantage of concrete is that it is easy to maintain and extremely durable. The disadvantage is that it must usually be installed by a contractor who either uses masonry blocks, hand-packed or poured concrete, or Gunite, which is a mixture of hydrated cement and silica sand.

A masonry spa can be relatively economical if it is constructed at the same time as the swimming pool it adjoins, and if it uses the same support system. But the majority of spas sold today are fiberglass shells. Fiberglass came into popularity in the 1960s as an alternative to hot tubs, and it offers an almost endless variety of shapes and sizes, although generally spas attain the same dimensions of 4' deep with a diameter of 4' or 5'.

The fiberglass shells normally have an inner lining made of acrylic or gelcoat. Acrylic is a hard, abrasion-resistant material that can readily withstand high temperatures and damage from chemicals. Gelcoat performs almost as well as acrylic, but it is easier to repair if its finish should in some way be damaged, and is considerably cheaper. In either case, the liner material together with the molded shell create a product that is only slightly more expensive than wooden hot tubs.

It is not very difficult to discern the quality of a wooden hot tub. All you need to do is look at the staves and note whether the wood grain is straight, vertical, and free of knots. Judging fiberglass and acrylic or gelcoat is nearly impossible. You can look at the thickness of the shell to be sure it is uniform by sighting along the surface. You can make certain there are no cracks or creases in the material. A good mold should be reinforced around the steps and all outlets, as well as across the bottom. But your best guarantee of workmanship is the reputation of the manufacturer.

The real difference in cost between hot tubs and spas comes with their installation. Fiberglass spas are not self-supporting in most cases, so they must be completely surrounded by some form of buttressing, which usually takes the form of sand. If the spa is placed in the ground, a hole is dug for the shell and then backfilled with well-tamped wet sand. If the unit is an above-grade installation, it must be surrounded by concrete or masonry blocks and still backfilled with wet sand. Either way, the digging and masonry work become an expensive—or if you do it yourself, time-consuming—process. Contractors charge in the neighborhood of $1,500 to $2,000 to install an average-sized spa.

THE COST OF OPERATION

Both hot tubs and spas must have an attendant support system comprised of water pumps, piping, and a hot water heater. Heaters are most often operated by natural or propane gas, although electric heaters are not uncommon. Better than either gas or electric from a maintenance cost point of view is a solar hot-water heating system, but solar is not widely employed as yet.

The cost of operating either a tub or a spa will quickly show up in your monthly electric and gas bills. You can assume that the cost of natural gas will be a shade less than electricity, and either source of heat will add twenty to twenty-five dollars a month to your utility bill. Add to that the cost of running the pumps, blowers, and lights and you can reckon another five dollars a month in electricity. There is also a monthly expense of ten to twenty dollars for chemicals to keep the water in proper condition. In other words, there is an operating cost of approximately fifty dollars a month for either a hot tub or a spa.

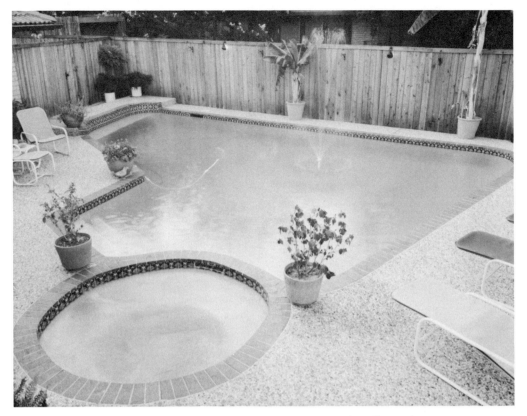

Spas are often constructed as adjuncts to a swimming pool.

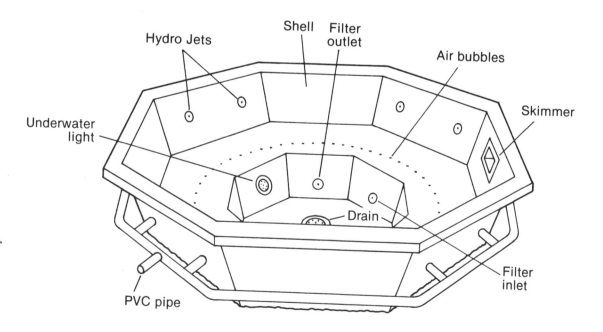

Anatomy of a fiberglass spa.

CHAPTER ELEVEN

Locating Hot Tubs and Spas

Before you even decide whether to have a hot tub or a spa, you ought to have some notion about where you will put such an object, and how it will look once it is installed. For the sake of your property and its appearance, your first expectation should be to have something that looks a little more interesting than an old wooden vat standing in the middle of the back yard, or a fiberglass fish pond without any fish.

Either a hot tub or a fiberglass spa actually offers numerous possibilities for landscaping a part or all of your yard and incorporating some pleasing changes of level into your environment. But you have a variety of considerations to take into account before you begin spending money.

ZONING

Before anything, read your local zoning laws and building codes. You will need to know such things as the legal setbacks, that is, how close to your property line you are allowed to build any structure; height limitations that govern the height of a tub as well as surrounding fences, breezeways, and walls; and whatever other restrictions are placed on you by the building laws. For example, you may be required to have a

secure cover for your tub or spa to prevent small children from getting into the water when the tub is unattended by an adult.

INDOORS OR OUT?

You can build your hot tub or spa out in the open, or house it either in your home or a roofed portion of your property. There are excellent reasons for choosing either locale, but there are also inherent difficulties with each.

Indoors, the tub is available for use day or night, rain or shine, cold or warm. In some parts of the United States, prevailing inclement weather during the spring, winter, and fall practically demands that your tub or spa be housed so that you have some modicum of control over the environment. Then there is the factor of privacy and child safety. An indoor bathing room can be locked when it is not in use to prevent small children from wandering into the steaming water. And by having walls and a roof over your tub, the neighbors and passers-by will not be able to bear witness to your nakedness should you decide to do your bathing in your most natural state.

On the minus side, keeping a hot tub or spa in

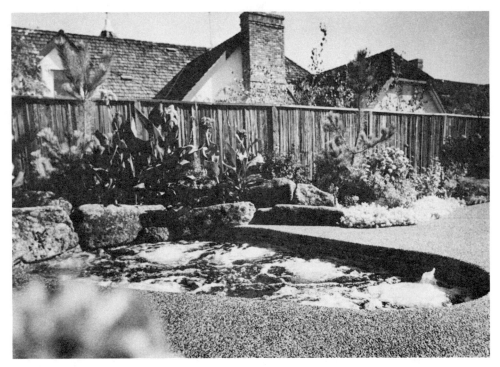

Before you install a hot tub or spa, have some idea about how it will look in its environment.

your house can cause a little extra thought and a lot of major construction problems. First of all, where do you put an object that is 5' across and weighs upwards of 5,000 pounds? If you already have a well-ordered home, just which room will you devote to the tub or spa? Unless your home happens to be of Buckingham Palace dimensions, there are not likely to be too many accessible but out-of-the-way nooks or crannies that can hold it.

Your purpose in having a tub in the first place is to provide a retreat of calm where you can relax. So the last rooms where you want to have your tub are the ones where people are always coming and going, or that are used as part of the daily traffic pattern. Moreover, you need to have the tub located near a dressing area so there won't be trails of water all over the house from the tub to wherever the bathers can change into their clothes. You might also consider locating the tub near the outdoors. Even if you have a stoop-sized patio outside a tiny window, it can enhance the pleasantness of your surroundings while you are soaking away the cares of the day.

After you have found a place in your house for the tub or spa, you have two complicated construction problems: weight and humidity.

WEIGHT

The floors in most houses constructed today are designed to support 40 pounds per square foot. A standard hot tub full of water and a couple of bathers can weigh over 250 pounds per square foot. You don't just shore up the joists with that kind of weight. You re-engineer the floor, the space beneath it, and probably will wind up replacing part of the concrete floor in your basement with a thicker, reinforced concrete slab.

Exactly what you have to do to accommodate your indoor hot tub or spa is probably spelled out in your local building code. Those accommodations will include provisions for the tub's foundation, its plumbing and its wiring, as well as proper ventilation. One of the requirements is likely to be that the floor under the tub must slope, and it must be made of water-resistant materials such as tiles, vinyl, or masonry. All four walls and the ceiling of the room that holds the tub must also be insulated and have a proper vapor barrier to resist moisture.

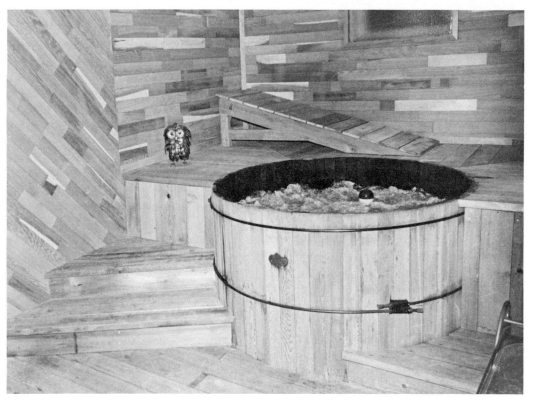

An indoor hot tub is available to you no matter what the weather is like, or the time of day or night.

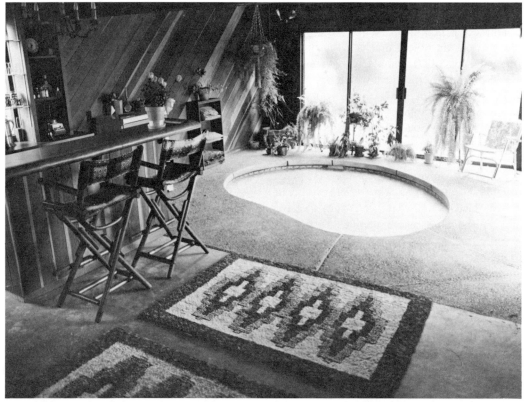

Deciding where a hot tub or spa can be placed in your house takes some extensive planning.

HUMIDITY

The primary defense against the tremendous amount of humidity that 500 gallons of hot water can give off to the air in any house is cross-ventilation. Condensation can—and will—collect on the ceilings, the walls, and windows, even when the tub or spa is not turned on. The ventilation system begins with a carefully designed cross-ventilation system throughout the house, but this may have to be supplemented with a forced-air system. In addition to this, such things as double-glazed windows and skylights that inhibit condensation, as well as moisture-loving plants, can be useful for controlling humidity.

PLANNING AN OUTDOOR SITE

The easiest way to find an appropriate outdoor location for your tub or spa is to use a sheet of ruled graph paper. On the paper accurately locate:

1. The dimensions of your lot.
2. Position the house, noting doors and windows, and the rooms they open into.
3. The four points of the compass (north, east, south, and west).
4. The path of the sun over the lot. Note any hot spots the sun creates on your property during the day.
5. Any water, gas, sewer, or electrical lines (as well as heating oil tanks) that are underground but might affect your installation.
6. The setback boundaries, which you can determine by asking your local building department for its setback limitations.
7. The direction of the prevailing winds during the winter and summer.
8. Any existing structures, including outbuildings, fences, gardens, patios, etc.
9. All existing plants and trees.
10. Note anything beyond your plot that might affect the tub or spa location. Unsightly buildings, for example, a neighbor's house, overhead utility lines, and so on.
11. If your lot slopes or is particularly irregular, you might consider doing a second drawing showing the slope in cross-section.

When you have completed your plot map, lay a piece of tracing paper over it and start sketching your notions about where the tub or spa should

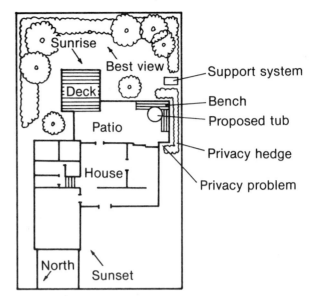

Lay out your property and everything on it on a piece of graph paper.

be situated. As you experiment, keep in mind such things as the ease of construction, traffic patterns that will develop around the finished installation, the visual effect of gardens, fences, and whatever else you will be able to see from the tub. When you have arrived at the area you think is best for the tub or spa, you can begin to evaluate some of your construction problems.

GRADE LEVELS

If you have a more or less flat plot of land where you can install your spa or hot tub you are blessed with the simplest and therefore least expensive possible installation. The ground can be hollowed out to accept a concrete slab or piers to support a hot tub with relative ease. It can also be dug out to hold an in-ground spa without any unusual problems.

It should be noted that trying to bury a hot tub is not something most people want to tackle because you have to dig two holes and line them with concrete, one to hold the tub and another larger sump to drain the water in the tub. In the bargain, you must also make sure that there is plenty of space around the tub so that air will flow freely enough to prevent the constant humidity from the hot water from rotting the wood in the tub. On top of all this, the pump-filter-heater support system must be kept aboveground

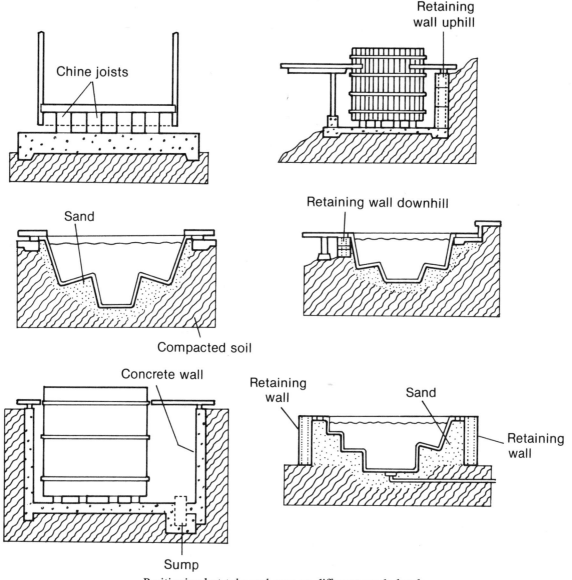

Positioning hot tubs and spas on different grade levels.

so there will be no risk of electrical short circuits should the pit around the tub ever flood.

If you are intent on burying your bathing equipment, opt for a fiberglass spa. It is easier to install below grade level. On the other hand, if you prefer an above-grade installation, it will cost you more to put in a spa than a hot tub. The reason for this is that spas must be surrounded by at least 9″ of sand on all sides. To contain that sand aboveground you cannot get away with loose earth, but must erect a solid masonry wall,

which of course will add to the cost of your construction.

In some ways, a sloping yard offers a maximum number of options so far as choosing between a spa or a hot tub. Essentially, to install a hot tub you will have to dig into the side of the slope and then place a concrete slab or piers. You may also have to erect a retaining wall on the high side of the excavation, but that is all. With a spa, you will still be able to dig into the slope, but may have to build up the low side with

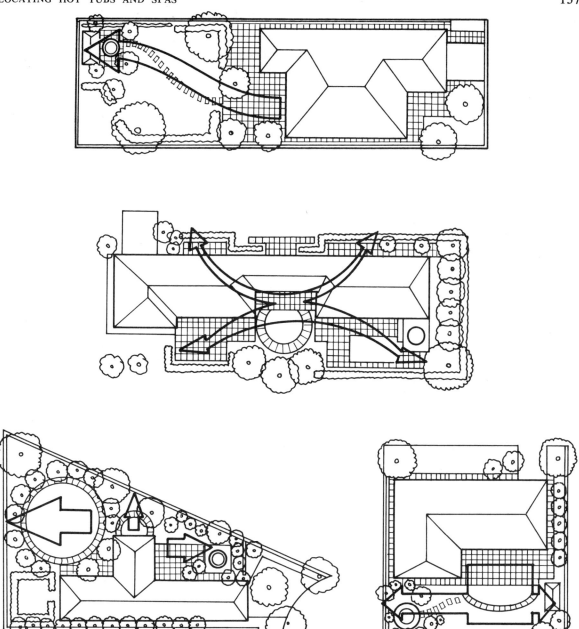

Some of the landscaping tricks used by professionals to minimize the shortcomings of different plots.

a retaining wall to support one or more sides of the unit. The amount of work needed and the cost of materials may, in the final analysis, be so close that you can decide on either the tub or the spa based on other considerations.

LANDSCAPING

You can look around your yard and see it as nothing but a liability that neither you nor anybody else can ever do a thing to improve. You can also see it as a challenge, particularly if it happens to be odd-shaped, or lumpy, or just plain awkward. There are no hard and fast rules you can apply to a plot of land in order to make it both functional and attractive. Because there are no rules you can let your imagination be your primary guide and do just about anything that appeals to you.

There are a few general comments that might be kept in mind as you work out what to do with the space around your hot tub or spa.

If you have a square lot, it presents a series of sharp angles not only in itself but in relation to the house, which is likely also to be very angular. You can make the lot look longer by establishing focal points at the corners—a hot tub in one corner, perhaps, a circular garden or small greenhouse in another, a stand of trees in another, some shrubbery in the fourth.

A wedge-shaped lot presents some sharp, narrow angles and the spaces between them are likely to be unequal. Again, the corners can be softened by filling them with trees, shrubbery, or gardens that offer more curves than angles. You might use one of those corners to shelter your tub or spa under a stand of trees. In between the corners, you might try to establish generous spaces of lawn or a small patio.

Shallow lots can be given a feeling of greater depth by creating focal points along the lot line with walkways curving away from the house that lead to plantings, or a patio, or isolated living

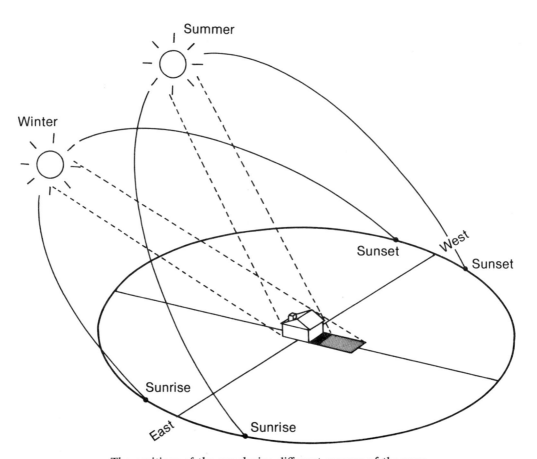

The positions of the sun during different seasons of the year.

areas such as a hot tub or a barbecue.

You can do things like turning an ugly outcropping of rocks into a rock garden, or lining a low, marshy area with plastic sheeting and turning it into a shallow pool where you can grow water plants. But whatever you do, please yourself. After all, you're the one who has to look at it every day.

BE AWARE OF THE CLIMATE

Before you situate your tub or spa, in fact even before you settle on where you will place it, take into account exactly what the climate around your house is all about. Consider the position of the sun over your property during the different seasons of the year; evaluate the prevailing breezes during both the winter and the summer.

Old Sol

The sun rises in the east and sets in the west—more or less. During the winter, it actually travels more from the southeast to the southwest, providing about nine hours of daylight from a comparatively low altitude. The result is that if you put a tub on the north side of your house, it will practically always be in the shade, which is fine if you live in a hot climate and want to protect the tub from hot summer rays.

During the summer, the sun rises more from the northeast and sets in the northwest, and provides around fifteen hours of hot sunlight daily. A tub at the north end of your house will still not receive full solar intensity, so if you live in a temperate or cool climate, you might be better advised to install it on the south side of your home where it can get the maximum benefits of the sun.

Only during the spring and fall does the sun actually rise in the east and set in the west, and during both seasons it will deliver twelve hours of daylight. A tub or spa situated on the eastern side of a home will have solar warmth only during the mornings; one on the west side of the house begins to receive direct sunlight by 11 A.M. and will continue to receive it all afternoon until sunset.

If you have a choice about where to place your spa or tub, then consider your living pattern. Will you be more likely to use it only in the mornings, or during the afternoons? Or do you need the tub to be protected from a fierce sun? Or would it be nice to have sunlight playing across the tub all day long?

Wind Patterns

The wind swirls around and over your house and land nearly every day, although it is likely to come from different directions during the hot and cold times of the year. If a great deal of wind blows over your tub or spa, it can make a cool day into a cold, uncomfortable time for bathing. Conversely, no wind on a steamy day can make bathing in a hot tub practically unbearable.

Too much wind around a hot tub can spray dust into the support system and evaporate, as well as cool, the water, causing the machinery to work harder than necessary. So the wind is a factor to be dealt with, and if necessary, modified.

You can deflect a prevailing breeze with shrubbery, but a better control is some form of fence made of wood, plastic, bricks, masonry, or glass. Essentially, a solid wall or fence standing in the way of a prevailing breeze will deflect the wind for a distance equal to the height of the barrier. Thus, a 6′ high fence will provide protection for about 6′ behind it. After that distance, the breeze dips sharply toward the ground again.

You can extend the effectiveness of the fence by tilting its top portion toward the wind. This will provide effective protection for a distance behind the fence that is equal to twice the height of the barrier. The baffle can also be angled about 45° in the direction of the tub behind the fence. This will prevent the wind from dropping sharply beyond a distance equal to the height of the fence.

Don't be fooled by the idea of an open fence. These have laths that are spaced about ½″ apart and while they do break the wind flow, dense shrubbery would provide considerably more shelter.

GIVING YOUR TUB OR SPA A PROPER SETTING

Whether you install a hot tub or a spa in-ground or at grade level, it needs to be given a visual setting that is both attractive and functional, which is why you always see pictures of decks and patios and gardens surrounding tubs and spas.

You must first decide, of course, whether you want the spa or hot tub to be a focal point of your plot or not. You have the option, in most situations, of making it either a major focal point

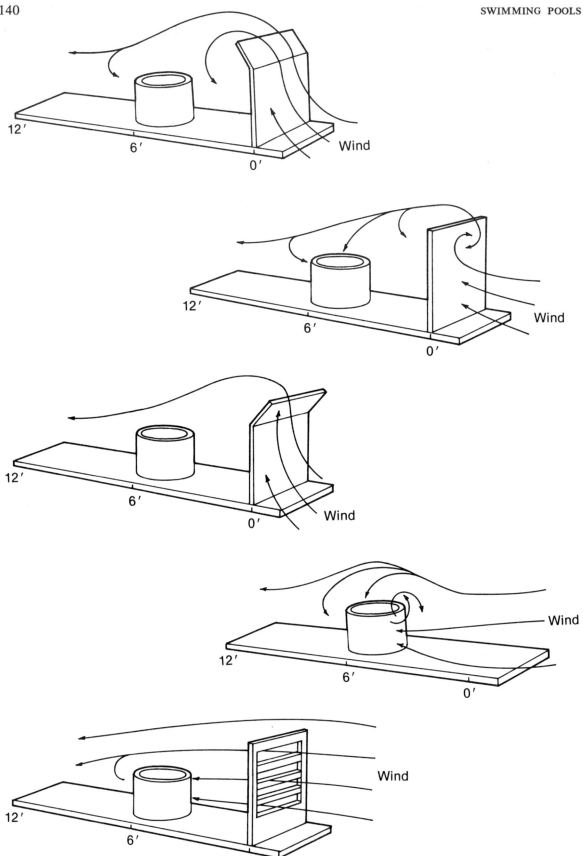

How the breeze reacts to different wind barriers.

or blending it into the environment so that it presents a more subtle element in your landscaping. Consider whether an aboveground hot tub will complement or vie with your patio or garden, swimming pool or deck. Do you want it to blend, or clash, with the architectural style of your house and the design of your garden?

If you elect to make the tub a focal point of your yard, you might want to frame it with benches and tiered decks, or surround it with shrubbery and plants. To achieve a more subtle effect, or to integrate the bathing unit with a swimming pool, you will need to surround it with flush paving or decking and soften its presence with plantings.

SHELTER

There are no rules that demand that any tub or spa be left uncovered to the elements. If you live in a warmer climate, you may find no reason to roof over the top of your spa or tub, since even bathing in the rain can provide its own sort of pleasures. But if the sun is overly fierce where you live, or if the winters are cold or dank, you may find advantages in building some sort of roof over your tub or spa. The ultimate shelter is, of course, a whole building constructed around the unit. Short of a complete structure, you can provide a lath roof, which will offer partial respite from the elements. You can use tempered glass or plastic sheeting, or build a lattice frame to support climbing plants.

The only rules that you need to follow when giving your hot tub or spa its own setting, whether it consists of patios or decking, gardens, windscreens, roofing, or just plain landscaping, are the rules that limit your imagination.

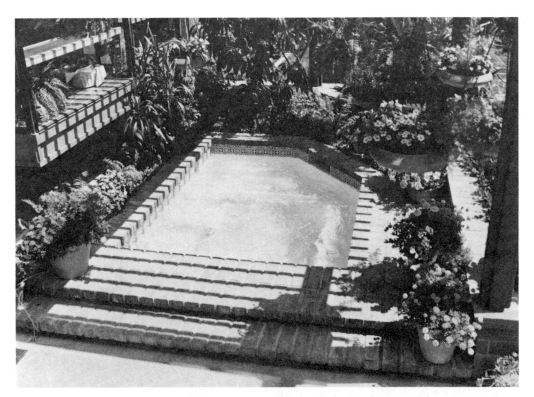

A spa or hot tub can be tucked into its surroundings, where it becomes a subtle accent.

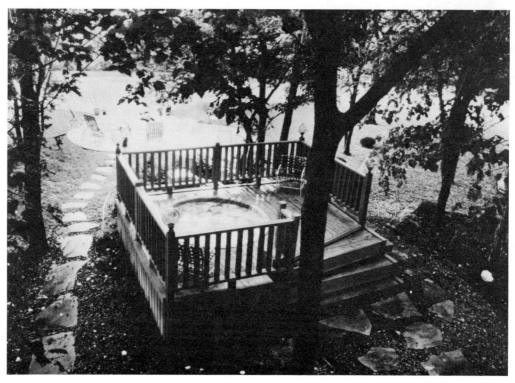

You can also make a spa or hot tub a focal point of your property.

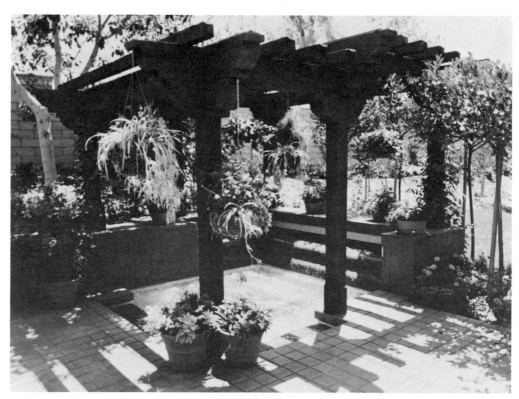

One way of sheltering a spa or hot tub without completely roofing it is to provide a lath roof.

CHAPTER TWELVE

Tub and Spa Support Systems

The support system for any hot tub or spa begins with its primary pump. The pump must be large enough to produce a high rate of water flow through the entire plumbing system. At the same time, you cannot have a pump that has a greater or a lesser capacity than the filter or heater, or the entire support system will be unbalanced and not work efficiently. So, before you install any support system, be sure that its components are balanced and have compatible capacities. To this end, you can purchase assembled components from a single manufacturer, or connect different units together into your own system.

THE PRIMARY PUMP

There is a myriad of centrifugal pumps available on the market at prices that range from $200 to $400. The centrifugal pumps used in tubs and spas are commonly ¾ to 2 horsepower and are capable of moving 50 to 105 gallons per minute *at level*. *At level* means horizontally. For every foot the pump must raise an amount of water, the gallons per minute drops considerably. While you can wire some centrifugal pumps for 120 volts, in most every instance the recommendation will be for 220 volts.

The pump itself consists of a motor that drives an impeller, or fan. The impeller sucks water past it and "impels" it through a pipe positioned in front of it at a high rate with low pressures. Pumps are available in brass, bronze, or plastic. The metal units are considerably more expensive, but they will last for as long as twenty years. The plastic versions are not quite as durable, but then they never corrode, either. If you opt for a plastic pump, understand that the unit must in some way be protected against freezing and overheating.

FILTERS

As soon as the tub water is drawn through the centrifugal pump, it is sent through a filter, which traps all solid materials in the water, purifying it. There are three types of filters used with hot tubs and spas, diatomaceous earth (DE), cartridges, and sand.

Diatomaceous earth (DE) is the most expensive type of filter, but it provides the tightest filtration. DE is a fine, chalky material which, when it is forced against permeable plates inside the filter housing, will trap just about any solid in the water, no matter how small it may be. A 50-

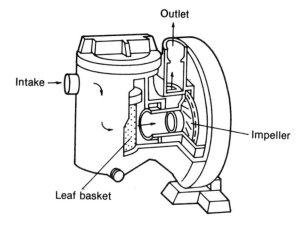

The primary pump.

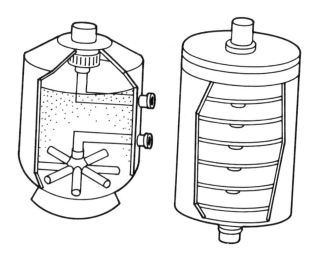

The sand filter (left) and the DE filter (right).

gallon-per-minute (gpm) DE filter costs between $280 and $320.

Cartridges are the least expensive, and provide the coarsest filtration. The cartridge contains rigid frames that hold liners made of Dacron, polyester, or some form of treated paper. The liners catch a lot of the solids in the water, but not all of them, so they must be replaced every two years or so. Fifty-gallon-per-minute capacity cartridges cost between $200 and $220.

Sand comes in a container that is about the same size as a DE filter and will do a filtering job that is somewhat better than cartridges and not quite as good as DE. A 50 gpm sand filter costs between $260 and $300.

HEATERS

From the filter the water passes through a heater, which can be fueled by natural or propane gas, electricity, heating fuel oil, or the sun. For most people today, the choice of heater depends more on the economics of the fuel it uses than on the design of the heater itself; you obviously want to select a heater that uses the least expensive fuel in your vicinity. In all cases, solar heating your hot tub or spa will be the least expensive to operate, and a proper solar heating arrangement can generate between 70 and 100 percent of your hot water needs. However, the installation cost of a solar hot water heating system is higher than any of the conventional heaters, plus the fact that most local building codes demand that any solar arrangement must also have a backup heating device. Which means you will have to purchase a conventional heater anyway, whether you use it or not.

OPEN-FLAME HEATERS

The heaters used with hot tubs and spas divide into three basic categories no matter what fuel they consume—coil, tank, and convection. *Coil heaters* permit a small volume of fast-moving water to pass near a large open flame, with the result that they can heat all the water in your tub in relatively quick order. Coil heaters are rated between 85,000 and 200,000 BTU's capacity and they consume a considerable amount of fuel, but for a relatively short period of time.

Tank heaters allow a large volume of slow-moving water to pass over a small flame and are rated at 20,000 to 40,000 BTU's. They cost less than coil heaters, but they require a long time to get the water up to its desired temperature and they tend to be inefficient in cold climates where the tub water may have gotten well below the normal 100° F. to 104° F.

Convection heaters are a combination of the coil and the tank heaters. They use a large coil to heat slow-moving water, which makes them the least expensive to buy and operate. Better yet, because of their slowness, you can use less powerful pumps and other support equipment. The rap against convection heaters is that they are very slow to heat the tub water during the last few degrees.

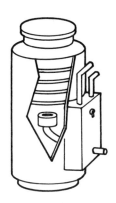 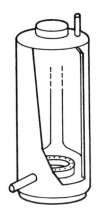 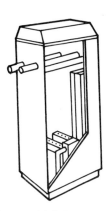

A convection heater (left), a flash heater (center), and tank heater (right).

ELECTRIC HEATERS

Convection, tank, and coil heaters can be purchased for use with natural or propane gas or home heating oil, but electrically powered heaters are a little different, since electricity does not produce an open flame. The electric heaters available perform much the way small tank heaters do but are comparatively slow, particularly if the whole tub has gone cold and all 500 gallons must be brought up 30° or 40°. Electric heaters are normally wired for 220 volts and are rated between 6Kw and 12Kw, which is the equivalent of 20,000 to 40,000 BTU's.

SOLAR HEATING ARRANGEMENTS

A solar heating arrangement can be adapted to your hot tub or spa and while it is not complicated to install and will operate virtually for the cost of electricity to operate its low-voltage pumps, it represents a large initial investment.

A swimming pool solar heating system requires inexpensive unglazed collector panels and PVC piping because the water in a swimming pool rarely needs to be heated by more than a few degrees. But a solar hot water heating system capable of delivering water at temperatures of 100° F. or more is, in effect, a scaled-down domestic hot water heating system. To heat an average hot tub or spa, you must have between 80 and 120 square feet of glazed collectors. Because of the heat of the water, the piping must be copper, rather than less expensive PVC plastic pipe. Water circulating out of the tub emerges from

the filter, and is pumped up to the panels through the collector loop, flows through the piping in the panels as it is heated by the sun's rays, then flows down to a conventional heater which will automatically raise its temperature if it is below the preset level of 100° F. to 104° F., before sending it back into the tub.

The solar heating system operates with a series of solenoid valves placed in the pipes between the collectors and the heater. The solenoids are commanded to open or close by a differential thermostat which is constantly comparing the temperatures of the water at both the panels and the cooler water coming out of the tank. If the tub water is hotter than the water in the panels, the thermostat automatically opens or closes the solenoid valves and diverts the water away from the panels, so that it will not overheat.

Although they sound complicated, solar heating arrangements are not difficult to install. The problem with them is their installation cost of $2,500 to $3,000 *plus* the cost of a backup heater. You cannot have just any little electric heater, either. Experts strongly recommend a large, fast recovery gas heater that can deliver 100,000 BTU's or more so that you are equipped to bring the temperature of the tub water up to its desired level quickly.

It is possible that with a solar heating system operating six hours a day, you may never need the auxiliary heater, and presuming you use your hot tub or spa during most of those hours, the system will pay for itself in a couple of years in terms of fossil fuel (gas, oil) that you do not

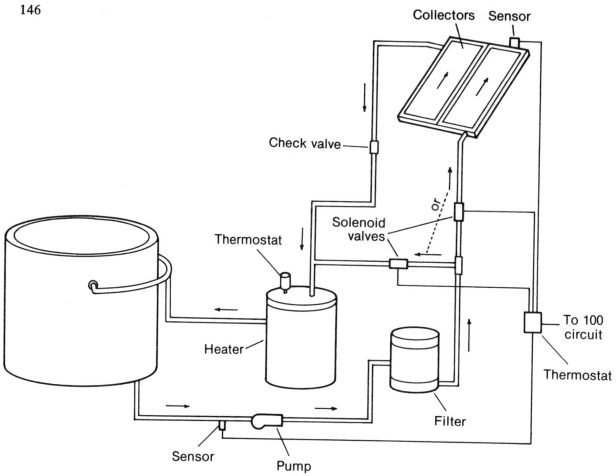

A typical solar heating system used to heat a hot tub.

have to purchase. But if you are only an occasional tub user, it could take as much as twenty years to retrieve the installation cost of a solar heating system.

The inclusion of a solar heating system in hot tub or spa installations is gaining in popularity, particularly in sunny climates and as the prices of gas, oil, and electricity continue to climb. But the choice depends entirely on your willingness and ability to withstand an added $2,500 or so to your initial installation costs. At least part of your decision to include a solar package should be made based on how quickly the investment can be recouped in terms of fossil fuel that does not have to be purchased.

JETS AND BLOWERS

The primary pump moves the water from the tub, through the filter and heater, and back to the tub. But in most instances, it is drawing water from the bottom third of the tub, so there is no sensation of water movement. In order to create the feeling of moving water, the pump must be boosted by one or more hydro jets and/or a blower.

Hydro jets, popularly known as venturi jets, are designed to restrict the flow of water through a small tube that consequently increases its velocity. The jets are affixed to the side of the tub near the surface of the water and some versions have an air intake, which produces bubbles in the water as it flows back into the tub. Many jets are also blessed with a swivel eyeball so that you can change the direction of the water flow.

Blowers can be attached to the hydro jets to increase the amount of air mixing with the water and therefore increase the bubbles in the tub. Blowers are normally operated separately and have their own switch. They must be installed at

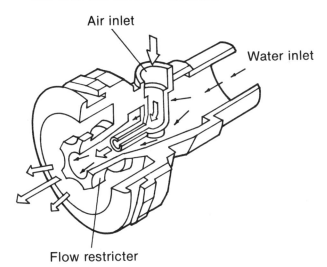

Air inlet

Water inlet

Flow restricter

Anatomy of a venturi jet.

least a foot above the water level or must be protected by an air loop or check valve.

THE UTILITY LINES

The pump, heater, filter, jets, and blowers are all connected to the hot tub or spa with both plumbing and electrical lines. When you install a hot tub or spa, you must first acquire all of the proper building permits from your local building department. Among those permits there will be one covering the plumbing and another that sets forth the standards to be met by all of the electrical work. Consequently, all plumbing and electrical work must meet industry standards of both workmanship and the kinds of materials used.

PLUMBING

There are likely to be four kinds of piping and fittings used to heat your hot tub or spa. *Copper* pipe and tubing are the traditional materials and they must be sweat soldered together in accordance with good plumbing practices. Copper is particularly used to construct the collector panel loop in solar domestic hot water installations and it will serve you for as long as the tub or spa is in use. It should be noted that copper transfers its heat very readily so it is best to wrap it in a good pipe insulation. Copper also must be used as a heat sink connection between most heaters and any plastic pipe used in the plumbing system.

Polyvinyl chloride (PVC) is the most commonly used pipe serving hot tubs and spas because it is lightweight, inexpensive, and easily assembled with a special cement. The major drawback to PVC is that it cannot withstand extreme heat or cold. In freezing weather, it becomes so brittle that it can crack. A better choice all around is chlorinated polyvinyl chloride (CPVC), which is manufactured specifically for use in hot water supply lines. In situations where a flexible tubing is needed, polyethylene (PE) is equally acceptable. In fact, many building codes prescribe the use of CPVC and PE over PVC.

The building codes also have some strict rules about the gas lines serving gas heaters. The pipe used for gas lines is always *black iron,* but the threaded connections in iron pipe must be carefully made or the gas will leak through them. Aside from the problems of renting, or the expense of buying, a set of dies to thread the lengths of pipe, you may be inhibited by your local code, which likely states that all gas connections must be made by a licensed plumber. You will probably have to hire a plumber to install the heater portion of your hot tub or spa.

The final alternative in piping is *galvanized steel.* Galvanized has been used in house water supply systems for years, but it presents many of the same difficulties in assembly as black iron in that the lengths of pipe must be cut, then threaded, then put together. Standard plumber's pipe dope or Teflon tape can be used to make your connections watertight, but there is still the hard labor involved with cutting the threads. It is considerably easier to use copper.

ELECTRICITY

The electrical connections that must be made in a hot tub or spa supply system include wiring the main pump, the air pump(s) if there are any, the heater, and any lights that may attend the installation.

An electric heater demands 220 volts and must be placed on its own circuit terminating at the house distribution panel. Because the heater is in the vicinity of water, the National Electric Code, and probably your local electrical code, demands the circuit breaker for the heater circuit to be a Ground Fault Circuit Interrupter (GFCI). Most primary pumps must also be wired for 220 volts

148

SWIMMING POOLS

and placed on their own separate circuit with a GFCI. Blowers and lights are normally rated for 115 volts and if they are not given a circuit of their own, they can usually be placed on an existing line. But no matter how they are wired, the circuit must also be protected by a GFCI.

Bear in mind that you are running electrical wiring to and around a vat filled with water, and electricity and water combined can become extremely hazardous to the health of human beings. It is absolutely mandatory that all electrical connections be properly made in accordance with local codes and the NEC, and that they be protected by Ground Fault Circuit Interrupters. The GFCI's are expensive (thirty to forty dollars each) but they are designed to react within a fortieth of a second to shut off the circuit should any electricity leak from it. They may not keep you from getting a mild shock, but they will most probably save your life in the event of a short circuit in any of the electrical systems while you are in the tub.

THE BASIC SUPPORT SYSTEM

The basic support system for an average-sized hot tub or spa employs a ¾ to 1 hp primary pump. The pump has a capacity that is compatible with a 50 gpm filter and a gas-fired coil heater delivering between 100,000 and 145,000 BTU's. The filter could be either a cartridge or a DE type. The number of jets you attach to such a system depends on the horsepower of the primary pump; a ¾ hp pump can handle two jets and a 1 hp pump is capable of handling three. If the pump is 1½ hp, you can add as many as five jets, but to handle six jets the pump must be increased to a full 2 hp.

However, when you change the pump size, you have to adjust the capacity of the filter as well. Up to 1 hp, the primary pump needs only a 50 gpm filter. At 1½ hp the filter must be increased to a capacity of 70 gpm; a 2 hp pump requires a 100 gpm filter.

The heater is not related to the primary pump or the rate of flow as much as it is to the jets and blowers. The number of jets and the presence of a blower can affect the recovery time of the heater since the blower (and the jets for that matter) speed heat loss from the water by making it move faster as well as adding air to it.

In most instances, your choice of heater will be based on recovery speed, that is, the time it takes for the unit to heat all of the water in your tub or spa. A 145,000 BTU gas-fired coil heater can heat a 500-gallon tub in a little over two hours, raising the temperature of the water from 50° F. to 104° F. A 12Kw electric heater needs five hours and an 85,000 BTU tank heater can do the same job in just under four hours. The quickest of all heaters is a 175,000 BTU coil heater, which needs about an hour and a half to heat an average 500-gallon tub or spa.

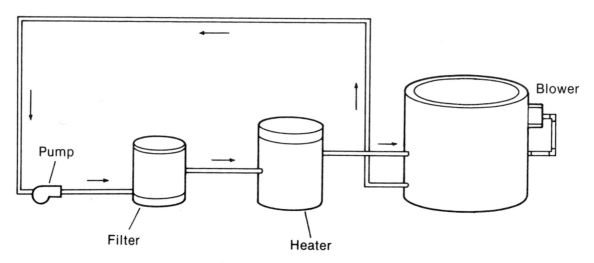

How the support system is interconnected with a hot tub.

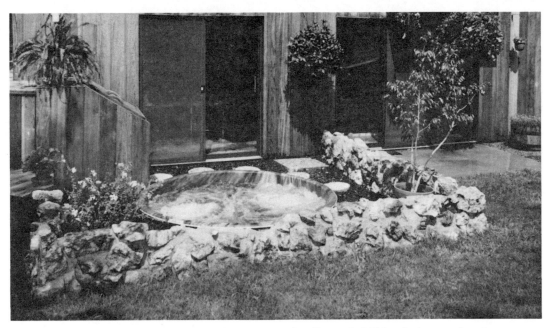

The support system for a hot tub or spa can be discreetly hidden in its own housing.

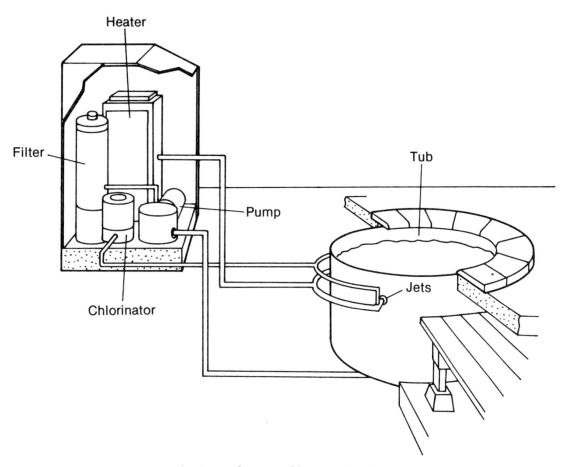

Anatomy of a spa and its support system.

EXTRA EQUIPMENT

There are two or three other devices that you might want to consider for use with either a hot tub or a spa:

Chlorinators. These are installed as a link between the inlet and outlet lines so that the disinfectant can mix completely before the water returns to the tub. Some units are semi-automatic and release the chlorine at a preset rate that can be manually adjusted. Completely automatic models dispense the chlorine on command from sensors, which are designed to adjust the flow continuously.

Automatic timers. These are twenty-four-hour clocks with on-off switches that can be set at different times of the day and night to start and shut off the primary pump and filter systems automatically. A coil heater can also be operated with a timer, but both tank and convection heaters must be operated by their own thermostats.

Pipe insulation. This is not expensive and can be purchased at any plumbing supply or home building center. The insulation is a sleeve that is wrapped around the pipes to be protected; this is useful if you live in a part of the country that has cold weather part of the year.

CHAPTER THIRTEEN

How to Build a Hot Tub

Considering the rising cost of both materials and labor, the idea of installing your own hot tub or spa offers the considerable appeal of as much as $1,000 in savings. On the other hand, you are taking on at least $1,000 worth of headaches and will devote at least that much in terms of your time and effort to complete the installation satisfactorily.

Manufacturer's installation guides for the particular tub and support equipment you buy tend to be twenty pages or more, which is not to say that any installation is complicated, only involved. Perhaps the first involvement to be considered is your local building code. In most parts of the United States, the local building code has specific demands concerning the installation of either a hot tub or a spa, beginning with the requirement that you have a building permit. You can probably "sneak" around the building code by ignoring it. But don't. The codes are your best guarantee that the job—whether you or a contractor does the work—is properly designed and is both operable and safe. If nothing else, when an installation meets all the code requirements, you can be assured that it is safe.

KITS

Some people buy a completed hot tub and then install it themselves. You can save considerable money by purchasing a tub kit, which includes floor joists, floorboards, precision milled staves, and metal hoops. The tools you need to assemble all this into a tub-sized vat are a rubber mallet, a brace of adjustable open-end wrenches, a drill, screwdriver, plane, and either a bench saw or a joiner-planer. You will also need some small nails, sandpaper, and perhaps some mastic, depending on the kit you have bought.

To get any hot tub kit assembled, you need two people. If the site of the tub happens to be a hard-to-reach location, you can make your life considerably easier by assembling the tub out in the open where you can move around it, and then finding a couple of extra people to help you carry it to its site. Putting a round tub together in tight quarters is asking for more trouble than it is worth, especially when four people can easily move the completed tub from wherever you put it together to wherever you intend to bathe in it.

152

STARTING ALMOST FROM SCRATCH

When you decide to construct a hot tub from a kit (you have to be an old-time cooper to start from scratch), the primary tasks you must complete are, in order: prepare the foundation to support the tub; construct the tub (unless you bought one already assembled); put up foundations for the support equipment; get the tub in place; and hook up all of the supporting equipment.

How you perform each of these tasks and the way each project looks when it is completed is dependent on an almost endless list of variables. The terrain and setting of your particular hot tub are most likely somewhat, if not totally, different from all other hot tubs. Then there are your particular construction skills, and the specific equipment you have elected to assemble into your hot tub system. The information that follows, therefore, is general in nature, and should be considered in terms of your particular circumstances.

FOUNDATIONS

The preferred foundation for any hot tub is a concrete slab, although in many cases you can get away with concrete piers on concrete footings. The reason concrete slabs are suggested by most manufacturers and installers is that they offer a total, level support for the tub, which prevents any unusual stress putting pressure on the tub itself. The piers, on the other hand, are nearly as stable a foundation, providing their footings are poured in well-packed soil.

Concrete Slabs

In order to hold the 5,000 or more pounds that a tub filled with hot water and people will weigh, the concrete slab under it should be a minimum of 4″ thick, and should be reinforced with steel rods. There should also be a footing at each corner of the slab as well as under its center portion. The footings should be at least 1′ deeper than the slab itself.

Dig down until you reach undisturbed earth and then level it. You should dig an extra 2″ below the thickness of the slab and fill the space with clean, well-tamped, leveled sand so that the slab can "float" in the earth and remain stable. If you are building the slab above ground level, you can construct the forms with 2″ × 6″ lumber braced with 1″ × 2″ or 2″ × 4″ support stakes placed no more than every 4′ apart. In either case, you actually want a 1″ to 1½″ tilt to one side of the tub so that it can drain should it overfill. Which side you tilt the slab to obviously depends on where you want any excess water to run; presumably you will not aim it at your house, but in some direction away from the building foundation.

You must also have a concrete slab and footings for the support equipment. This is normally a 3′ × 5′ area and in most cases need only be 3½″ thick. But check the size of your equipment to make sure 3′ × 5′ is an appropriate set of dimensions before you pour any concrete.

Bear in mind that concrete needs at least six days to cure properly, so do your slab work a

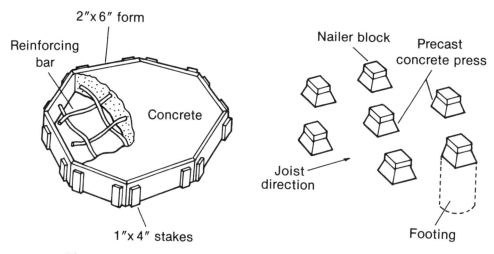

The foundation for a hot tub can be either a concrete slab or footings.

week or more in advance of when you plan to put the hot tub on top of it.

Footings and Piers

If you hire a contractor to install your hot tub, he may recommend against using piers. There is a possibility with piers that drainage or water running under the tub will cause the footings to settle unevenly. Actually, the subject is up for debate with as many experts claiming that piers and footings are just as reliable as slabs as there are people who abhor the use of piers.

The footings under each pier should be sunk several inches in packed subsoil and should also reside below the frost line; depending on where you live in the United States the frost line can be anything from 3″ to 24″ below the surface of the ground. According to common concrete and masonry practice, a pier footing should be the same thickness as the pier and twice the width. The piers themselves rise above ground level and are arranged in a pattern suggested by the tub manufacturer. This normally means four or five piers are placed around the perimeter and a center unit is built under the middle of the bottom of the tub. The pattern is designed to provide an even distribution of weight on each pier and also to locate the joists inside the inner circumference of the tub sides. The joists must also be oriented so that the drain line running to the pump does not require any elbows. The tops of the piers should be level with each other, but they can be sloped so that the joists angle about an inch in one direction to provide for any excess runoff that may occur.

THE ASSEMBLY

When the piers have been poured into their forms, anchor bolts must be embedded in their tops to hold nailer blocks. The blocks are drilled to accept the bolts and can be installed after the concrete has cured for six or seven days.

JOISTS

When the concrete has cured, joists are across the nailer blocks and toenailed to the piers. The primary concern at this stage is to make certain that all of the joists are level with each other and that the slope along each of them is identical. If you are required to shim any of the joists to align them properly, place the shims *under* the joists, between their bottom edge and the top of the nailer blocks. Do *not* put the shims on the top edge of the joist since they will cause parts of the tub to be unsupported.

FLOOR

The floor of the tub is designed to spread the weight of the unit evenly along each of the floorboards. To accomplish this, the floorboards may be either tongue-and-groove assembled or connected by dowels. As a further protection against excessive leakage when you first put water into the tub, some manufacturers recommend that you squirt a bead of mastic along the bottom edge (underside) of each board. It is essential that the mastic be kept along the bottom edge of the flooring so that as the boards swell and exert pressure, it is prevented from rising up to

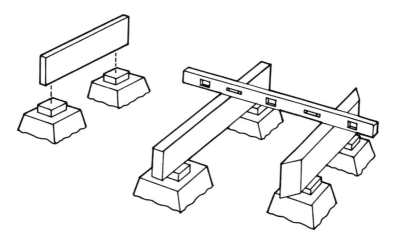

The joints are placed across the footings or bolted to the slab.

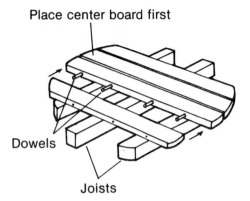

Place center board first

Dowels

Joints

The floor is assembled and placed on the joists but not anchored to them.

the inside of the tub, where it could leach chemicals into the bathing water.

To prevent leakage in the floor of the tub, you obviously do not want to nail any of the floorboards to the joists. Putting a nail through the wood is tantamount to boring a hole in the bottom of your tub. Consequently, the tub floor merely sits on its joists, but it must do so in such a way that the bottoms of the staves do not touch any of the joists.

The staves have a rout, or dado, cut out of them to accept the ends of the floorboards. The dado is a square trough milled out of the wood about an inch from the end of the stave, leaving the end, or chine, of the stave, comparatively weak. If the tub were allowed to stand on the bottoms of its staves, its weight would eventually cause the chines to break. In other words, the floorboards must extend beyond the joists in all directions.

When assembling the floor of the tub, begin by placing the center board across the joists and then hammer a board to each side of it with your mallet. Add boards alternately to opposite sides of the center board until the entire floor has been assembled. If you have assembled the floor somewhere other than over the joists, take it to the site and test fit it over the joists once it is completed. You want to be very sure that the chines will not rest on any of the joists.

STANDING THE STAVES

It is critical that all of the staves be given the proper spacing. Moreover, if the kit you are as-

sembling has some of its staves predrilled for the support system pipes, the drilled staves must be placed so they are aimed directly at the support system slab.

Prior to assembling the staves, the entire kit should be stored in a warm, dry place so that the wood is as close to the state it was in at the time it was put together at the factory. If, for example, the staves have been subjected to moisture prior to assembly, you may well find that the last stave must be shaved down before you can fit it into the tub.

Each stave must stand up vertically from the floor of the tub. The edge of the flooring is inserted far enough into the dado of the stave so that the stave can stand erect. Ultimately, when all of the staves have been assembled around the floor, they are tightened against the floor with the hoops, not by hammering them.

Many manufacturers suggest scribing a line around the edge of the floor that is the depth of the dadoes in the staves. For example, if the dadoes are ½″ deep, the line is scribed ½″ inside the edge of the floorboards. Once the line is drawn, you will be able to see when the bottom of each stave is fully seated on the flooring.

Under no circumstances do you want any of the joints between the staves to align with any joints between the floorboards. Center the first stave so that it is across one of the floor joints and tap it onto the edge of the boards until it is snug enough to stand up. Do not bang the stave more than half the depth of its dado.

Working clockwise around the tub floor, attach each of the remaining staves, tapping them halfway into their routs and seating them snugly against each other at their bottoms. They will stand at various angles away from each other at their tops, but they will all be brought together once you attach the hoops.

If, at some point, the joint between a pair of staves falls in line with one of the floor joints, you have two options. You can remove the last stave and continue erecting staves in a counterclockwise direction, then trim the last two staves so they meet away from the joint. Or you can try tapping the existing staves in one direction or the other until the last joint is a minimum of ⅛″ away from the floor joint. While it requires more work to move the staves, it is always safer to avoid trimming any wood if you can help it.

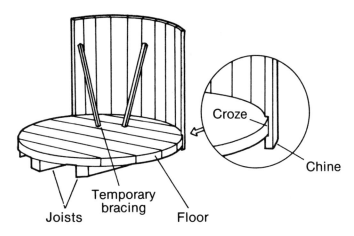

The staves are stood up around the perimeter of the floor.

If the last stave is too wide to fit, you may have no choice but to rip it down to size. You do this by measuring the gap between the staves at both their inside and outside edges and then cutting the last stave to your dimensions. The safest way of shaving down the stave is to use a joiner-planer. If you use a bench saw the blade must be set to the same angle as the sides of the stave and then used to rip the wood. It is better to bring the stave down to its required width with several passes of the saw than to try to take off exactly the right amount of wood with a single cut; if you make the stave too narrow, you will have to buy an extra stave and that may not fit either.

HOOPING IT UP AROUND YOUR TUB

When all of the staves are in place, they are brought snugly together by tightening rolled steel hoops around the outside of the tub.

All kit manufacturers have specific instructions for spacing the hoops, but the first one you attach is always the bottom one, and it is always positioned at the edge of the tub floor, across the back of the dadoes in the staves.

If you have not used an assistant so far when assembling your tub, you will need one now. It takes two fairly strong people to bend the hoop around your tank and thread the ends into their retaining lug. The lug can be centered over any of the stave joints, preferably somewhere out of the way of whatever traffic pattern will pass around the tub. Working clockwise, each succeeding lug should be positioned over a different stave joint.

The first step is simply to get the hoops wrapped around the outside of the tub and tightened until they are barely snug against the wood. In order to hold them in place, drive a small nail into every seventh stave all the way around the tub and rest each hoop in its respective nail line.

When all of the hoops are in place, one person gets inside the tub with a mallet and the other person works the lugs on the hoops with a pair of wrenches. At this point, the staves are still only partially seated over the tub floor; some of them will angle inward, others outward. Beginning with the bottom hoop, the inside worker taps the various staves, straightening them out as the outside man cinches the hoop. The work progresses upward from hoop to hoop, moving constantly around the tub until the bottoms of all the staves are aligned with the scribed line, and all the hoops are as tight as they can be made.

The tub is now ready to accept its plumbing connections and built-in seats, if there are to be any. If the tub has been built away from its site, it should first be placed on its joists.

PUTTING IN A SPA

Fiberglass shell spas require considerably fewer steps to install, but each stage must be exactly correct before you can go on to the next procedure. There are also comparatively fewer chances to correct an error than there are with wooden tubs.

To begin with, the spa comes in one large, awkward piece, which means that the most im-

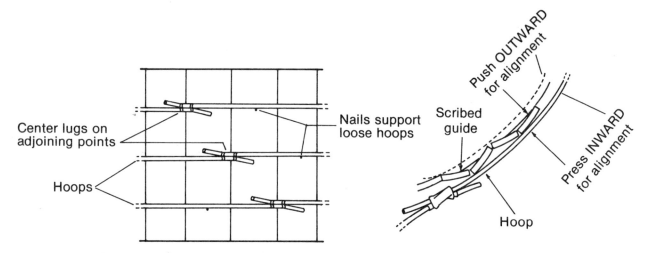

Center lugs on
adjoining points

Hoops

Nails support
loose hoops

Push OUTWARD
for alignment

Scribed
guide

Press INWARD
for alignment

Hoop

The hoops are placed around the staves and tightened until every stave is completely
seated on the edge of the floor.

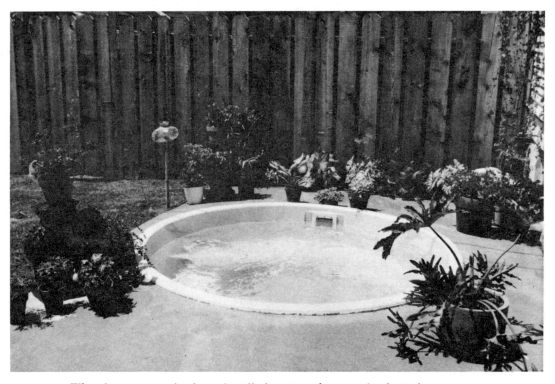

Fiberglass spas require fewer installation steps than wooden hot tubs.

portant part of its installation is preparation of the building site.

SITE PREPARATION

You can set a spa in the earth or stand it aboveground by building up masonry or concrete walls around it, but in either instance, your first task is to create a hole 6″ deeper than the spa and at least 9″ larger than its circumference. You also have to dig trenches for the plumbing, and bear in mind that the lip of a fiberglass spa cannot support any of its weight. The lip is supposed to be either recessed under the surrounding deck or fitted over the decking without bearing any of the weight of the tub. Consequently, before you place the shell in its hole, drive stakes into the ground at all four corners and nail 2″ × 4′″s between them, making the stringers absolutely level with the ground and each other. You can then rest the spa on the lumber and get it into its final position while the hole is being backfilled.

GETTING A SPA IN PLACE

Before you place a fiberglass spa in its excavation, assemble the main drain and the water line in the appropriate knockouts provided in the side of the shell. In practically every instance, the fittings are made by coating a gasket with sealant on both sides and then tightening lock nuts as hard as you can without using a wrench. If you put a pair of wrenches on the nuts, you may break the shell, so resist the temptation to crank them down as tight as you can get them. It isn't necessary anyway, if the gaskets are properly sealed.

With the drain line in position, lift the shell into its hole and rest it on the 2″ × 4″ stringers. If the drain line touches soil, dig out under it until there is ample clearance, then begin backfilling sand under the shell.

Actually there are two arguments about backfilling, so you take your choice. Some manufacturers and contractors insist that the best way

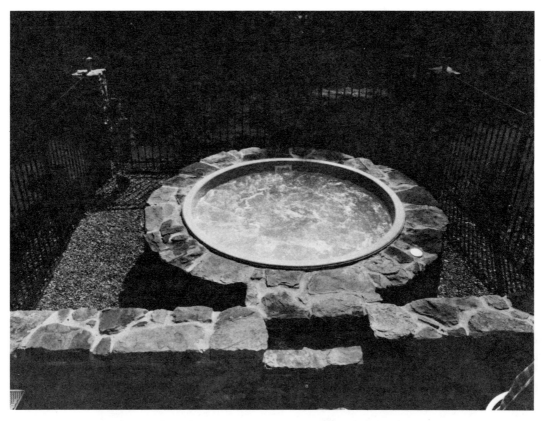

The lip of a fiberglass spa must not support any of the unit's weight.

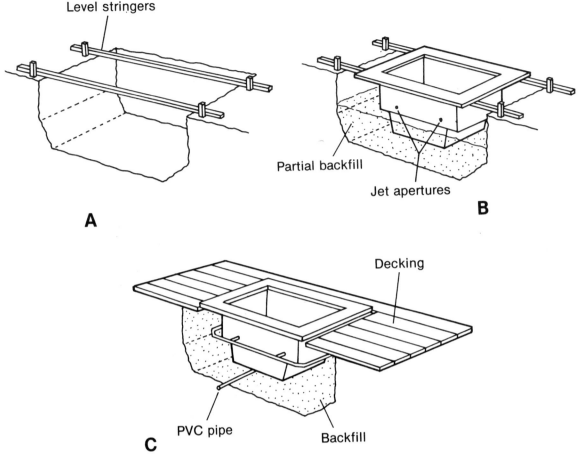

How a fiberglass spa is placed in its hole and backfilled.

is to cover the bottom of the hole with clean, well-packed, wet sand. The shell is then rocked down into the sand base until it has carved its own hole. The other approach is to hang the shell over its hole and shovel sand under it until all the spaces are filled. In either case, you have to fill in under the shell completely, leaving no air pockets in the hole.

There is also a mild debate over whether the sand should be just wet or whether it should be mixed in a ratio of 4 parts sand to 1 part portland cement. The addition of cement to the mix will create a solid plate of concrete to support the spa, but there is no guarantee that it will overcome the problem of erosion any more than well-tamped wet sand.

No matter how you backfill your excavation, the backfill continues up to the level of the drain in the side of the shell connections. At that point, the drain line must be laid before backfilling up as far as the second level of plumbing lines. Be certain that the lines have all been pressure connected, and that the shell is level and standing solidly before completing your backfill around the sides.

When the spa is completely situated in its excavation, the final stage is to construct the decking around the edges of the spa.

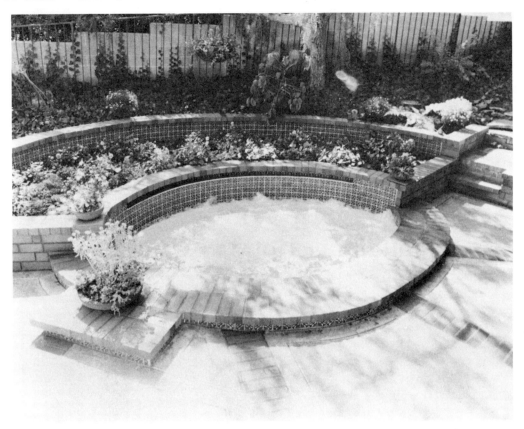

When the spa is in place, the final step is to complete the decking around it.

CHAPTER FOURTEEN

Maintaining Hot Tubs and Spas

When your hot tub or spa is completely installed and is apparently ready for use, it still isn't ready. There is yet another week or so of curing and conditioning the tub or spa before you can jump in and soak away all your cares and woes.

GETTING A HOT TUB READY

The first problem you will encounter with any wooden hot tub is that it leaks. The tub has been assembled by placing a series of curved wooden staves in a groove cut around the edge of a wooden bottom plate. The staves are held in place by iron hoops that are bolted with lags where their ends meet. If the tub was properly assembled, there are even spaces between each of the staves that will close once the wood has been soaked and had an opportunity to swell and become watertight. There is no caulking between the pieces of wood, nor does there need to be if the unit has been correctly constructed.

The first time you fill the tub, use a lawn sprinkler attached to the end of a garden hose. The sprinkler should be hung near the top of the tub and aimed in such a way that it can spray the in-

side of the staves as water fills the tub. In this manner, the wood will have an opportunity to begin swelling even before the tub is completely full, when it must support the full weight of 500 gallons of water. Even so, leaks will occur and continue for anywhere from a day to a week before the staves are swollen enough to become watertight.

CURING UNUSUAL LEAKS

A well-made tub will leak profusely between all or most of its staves at first and then gradually become watertight. But sometimes the tub has not been perfectly made, in which case you will have some repair work to perform.

If any of the initial leaks are more like gushes, either the staves have been milled improperly or they are poorly spaced. You can determine the milling by looking at the grain of the wood in the staves. It should be straight and run directly from top to bottom with no knots. If every stave is not like this, return the whole tub to the manufacturer and get a replacement.

Poor, uneven spacing between the staves can

be rectified by loosening the lugs on the hoops one or two turns, but no more than that. Begin at the staves on the opposite side of the tub from the leak, and use a rubber mallet to pound the staves into alignment. Hit the bottom of one or two staves on each side of your starting point. Then continue to alternately push the staves into alignment or make them tighter together on either side of your starting point until you have worked your way completely around the tub to the offending leak. Your objective is to even the spacing between the staves so that they all stand parallel to each other. When you are satisfied that you have accomplished this, tighten the lugs in the hoops.

If, after a week of soaking the tub, you still have some leaks, the most practical approach is to stuff cotton caulking string (known as rotten cotton) into the cracks, the way people caulk between the planks of a wooden boat. You can caulk from either the inside or the outside of the staves, although you will find arguments for and against whichever side you choose. The advantage of caulking from the outside is that you can see the leak and attack it directly by stuffing the caulking string into it, using a putty knife or spatula to seat the material well between the staves. The danger in caulking from the outside is that pressure from the water will be against the string and in time could conceivably push it out of place. If you caulk from the inside, the water pressure will only tend to drive the caulking string deeper between the staves. But then, if you caulk from the inside, you must first empty the tub and then locate the crack.

If a leak is coming from the bottom of the tub along the joint between the staves and the floor, the full weight of 500 gallons of water is pushing against the leak and the only way you can stop it is by caulking from the inside.

If you get a leak through one of the staves, the wood has a weak spot in it that cannot be caulked. It can be stopped, however, with a coat or two of marine (exterior) grade polyurethane varnish. Drain the tub to below the leak and allow the spot to dry. Then apply two or three coats of varnish. When the last coat has dried, fill the tub again.

Only in rare instances should you consider the use of any caulking other than cotton string. If the string has not stopped the leak, or if you are unable to get any string into a leaking joint, fill the crack with a plastic-based marine putty, but only apply it to the outside of the tub and don't use it at all unless you absolutely must.

BATHING IN TEA WATER

Unweathered redwood contains a considerable amount of tannin, a substance that is also found in tea. The tannin from redwood is as harmless as the tannin you consume every time you drink a cup of tea. And like tea, the tannin in redwood will give your bath water a lovely brown tint that will not disappear until all of the chemical has leached out of the wood.

There is no harm in tannin, but the color of it seems to bother most people when they bathe, so you will most likely want to clear up the color of your water. The recommended method of doing this is to fill the tub and let it get as dark as you can stand, then empty the tank. Do not turn on your filter during this period. Water with a heavy tannin content will strain the filter and render it useless.

Once you have gotten rid of the first tub of water/tannin, you can use the filter two or three hours a day in between frequent refillings and drainings of the tub. You will find that you can get a day or two of clear water after each refilling before more of the tannin darkens the water again.

You can also hurry the process of getting rid of tannin by chlorinating every other day, rather than once a week, until the tub water remains clear. It should be noted that most professionals no longer recommend putting soda ash in the tub during its first filling. It is true that a dose of 2 pounds of soda ash for every 1,000 gallons of water will help draw tannin out of the wood, but it will also damage the staves.

CRANKING UP THE SUPPORT SYSTEM

Your hot tub or spa support system is made up of three major pieces of machinery; each has its own set of rules so far as start-up and maintenance are concerned. Don't touch any buttons, levers, switches, or anything else until you read and understand all of the manufacturer's starting and maintenance instructions. These will, of course, vary according to the manufacturer, the model, and the unit itself, but there are two immutable laws that must be followed, whether you arm yourself with a full knowledge of the hardware or not:

1. Be absolutely certain the entire pump/filter system is fully primed before you turn on the primary* pump. That means all the air in the pump/filter system must be bled out of it and replaced with water.

2. Make certain the heater is full of water before you light any fires in it or turn it on, or you will burn out the unit almost immediately. This is especially true of electric heaters.

BASIC MAINTENANCE

The maintenance of any hot tub or spa divides into three distinct operations: Keeping the water clean and augmented with the proper chemical content; keeping the surfaces of the tub or spa clean; and keeping the pumps, filters, and heater in proper working order.

CLEAN WATER

If you own a swimming pool, you already know about the problems of keeping the water in a large receptacle clear of algae and invisible bacteria. But with the hot water used in tubs and spas, the problems of maintaining clean water are multiplied, because human skin is especially subject to infection in hot water. Moreover, too many solids in the water puts an inordinate strain on the pump and the filter, and if that water is also chemically imbalanced, whatever metal is in your support system may begin to corrode.

High temperatures combined with bubbles in the water are an open invitation for both bacteria and algae to multiply at an astounding rate, particularly because heat and bubbles also tend to break down the disinfectant normally used to inhibit that growth. Add to this the fact that four or five people soaking in a tub give off considerable amounts of body oils, strands of hair, and modicums of dirt that are dutifully pumped into the filter (which means the filter must be tended to on a regular basis). Plus, high temperatures intensify the evaporation of water, which in turn speeds up the amount of mineral scale that accumulates in the support system and on the inside surfaces of the tub or spa. The upshot of all this

is that you have to pay regular attention to keeping the water in your spa or hot tub clean.

Water maintenance is not difficult, but it must be done regularly. And it begins with the filter, which must not only be kept clean itself, but used on an average of two to three hours a day. The real secret to keeping your water clean is to own—and use—a water test kit. The kit should be capable of testing four things:

1. Potential Hydrogen (pH)
2. Total alkalinity
3. Chlorine or bromine
4. Water hardness

You can buy a kit for as little as $5.00 or spend as much as $75. The more expensive ones typically include enough of a variety of corrective chemicals to last you several months. Each kit available on the market has slightly different testing procedures, which are detailed in its manufacturer's instruction manual; those procedures should be followed exactly for each test the kit is capable of making.

THE ESSENTIAL CHEMICALS

Most people use about the same chemicals to treat the water in their tubs or spas as are applied to swimming pools. But since tubs and spas are smaller and contain hotter water than pools, the chemicals must be handled somewhat differently. How differently can vary almost from owner to owner, since water varies so widely in chemical content from region to region. Nevertheless, the most usual chemicals employed are:

Chlorine or bromine. These are both disinfectants and should be injected into the water on a regular basis.

Soda ash. This is an alkali and is used to balance water that is overly acidic.

Water clarifier. Clarifiers tend to coagulate any microscopic solids in the water so they become big enough to be trapped in the filter.

Water softener. There are numerous types of water softeners, beginning with ordinary salt. The ones you use must be suited to the mineral content of the water in your tub or spa. The purpose of putting a softener in your tub or spa water is to minimize staining and mineral scale. The staining occurs on the wooden tub; the mineral scale will, in time, clog up the pipes and machinery in your support system.

Algaecide. This is used whenever the algae in

your water is too tough to be dissipated by chlorine or bromine.

Antifoam agent. This is an agent for getting rid of suds in water.

All the disinfectants are important for maintaining clean water in your tub or spa, but the essence of good water is to have the right potential Hydrogen (pH).

If the pH is over 7.8, it is said to be too high in pH and must be balanced by adding acid. If you neglect to treat a tub full of water that has an acid/alkaline imbalance, there are four problems that could arise:

1. The water may grow hazy.
2. The filter may clog.
3. Mineral scale may form on the sides of the tub or spa and, worse than that, on the insides of the support equipment.
4. The effect of whatever disinfectant you add to the water will be reduced considerably so far as its ability to inhibit the growth of both algae and bacteria.

Adding Acid

It is comparatively difficult to test water for acid content, so most people test for pH and correct their water by referring to a chart that is printed on the package of acid. Most dealers suggest a dry acid for use in tubs and spas because it is easiest and comparatively safest to use. The general procedure for adding acid to a tub or spa is:

1. Shut off the primary pump and keep it turned off until the acid has been completely mixed with the tub water to avoid concentrates of acid getting into the pump and filter.
2. In a pail, dissolve 1 ounce of dry acid in 2 gallons or more of water.
3. Partially submerge the bucket in the center of the tub or spa, well away from the sides of the unit. By submerging the bucket, the acid mixture will merge with the tub/spa water slowly.
4. Mix the acid mixture with the tub or spa water by turning on the blower if you have one, or stirring the water with a stick or paddle.
5. Only after the acid is thoroughly mixed can the primary pump be turned on.
6. Wait at least an hour before adding any chlorine to the water. If you add it any sooner than an hour you are running the risk of a dangerous interaction between the two chemicals.

If you own a swimming pool, you are used to treating the water with muriatic acid. Muriatic acid is *not* recommended for use in hot tubs or spas. In its concentrated form it is strong enough to damage the wood of a hot tub or etch the walls of a spa, particularly if the spa has fiberglass or gelcoat finishes. Moreover, if you splash the acid on yourself, it will burn your skin. If you do decide to use muriatic acid, dilute it in a pail and float it into the tub or spa *very carefully.*

Adding Alkali

When the pH is below 7.2, the water is too acidic and should be balanced by adding alkaline to the water. There are three possible results from water that has a low pH:

1. The water may cause irritation to human skin or sting human eyes.
2. Any metal touching the water will probably corrode, which means much of your support system may be in danger of coming to a halt.
3. The water may scar the finish on the inside of your spa; if you have a hot tub, it will break down the cell walls of the wooden staves and bottom plate.

The most common alkaline used by tub and spa owners is soda ash, although manufacturers sometimes recommend alternative chemicals. Whenever the pH is below 7.2, alkali should probably be added to the water. However, the pH measurement does not tell you how much acid or alkali is actually in the water. It merely tells you the balance between the two. Therefore, the water should be tested for alkali at least once a month, or anytime a high pH persists.

The accepted range of alkali is between 90 and 180 parts per million (ppm). If the alkaline content is less than 100 ppm, it is time to start adding soda ash. Or, if there is no water shortage in your area, drain off about half your bathing water and refill the tub or spa with fresh water.

If the test for alkalinity shows more than 180 ppm, the pH is most likely too high and you will have to correct for acidity.

Chlorine and Bromine

The most common disinfectant used to control bacteria is, of course, chlorine, but bromine is gaining considerable acceptance among spa and tub owners as a viable alternative. Chlorine can be purchased as a liquid, in granulated form, or as tablets. It is in its most caustic form as a liquid, making it difficult to introduce into the relatively small amounts of water found in tubs or spas without risking damage to the unit. It is most stable in its granulated form, which means that it will dissolve easily in the water and has been treated to lose a minimum of its effect from ultra-violet rays. As a tablet, chlorine can be injected into the tub or spa water with a chlorinator, which allows the disinfectant to mix thoroughly before it enters the tub water.

The usual method of introducing either disinfectant into your tub or spa is to dissolve granulated bits into a pail of 2 or more gallons of water, mix thoroughly, and then slowly submerge the pail into the tub or spa, keeping it as far away from the walls of the unit as possible. If there are high concentrations of organic material in your water, the bromine is considered more effective than chlorine, but in either case the prescribed proportion should be between 1.0 and 2.0 parts disinfectant per million. If the ppm is below 1.0, the disinfectant will be ineffective; over 4.0 it becomes an irritant to human skin and eyes. Moreover, an excess of chlorine can corrode the metal in your support system.

Testing for Disinfectants

You should test for both disinfectant and pH every second or third day, then correct the disinfectant first. One popular maintenance approach is to correct the disinfectant whenever it is low, to bring the level to a shade over 2.0 ppm. Then add a massive dose every two weeks to raise the ppm level to 6.0. Do not run your primary pump while the disinfectant is being added to the tub or spa water, and if you are adding a heavy dosage wait until the ppm level has settled back to the 2.0 to 4.0 range (in about an hour) before turning the pump on again. You can minimize the dissipation of the disinfectant by adding it after the sun has set or whenever the heater will not be in use for several hours.

Hard Water

The harder water is, the higher its mineral content. The minerals can be almost anything, depending on the region where you live, although most probably both calcium and magnesium will be present. No matter what minerals are in your water, they will increase as the water is heated and evaporates.

The kind of softener you use depends on the mineral content of your water. In general, a hard water should be treated so that the ppm count of softener chemical is as high as 1,000. Providing the water is also kept clean and in proper balance, a single filling of the tub should last from one to four months before the water must be changed.

SAFETY PRECAUTIONS WITH CHEMICALS

All of the chemicals needed to maintain the water in your hot tub or spa are concentrated and as such should be handled carefully. Some of them may explode if they are mixed together; others may give off dangerous gases. Whenever you are handling or storing chemicals, keep these rules in mind:

1. Never mix two chemicals together. Even divergent types of chlorine may cause a chemical reaction when mixed.

2. When you are diluting any chemical, never pour the water into the chemical. Always pour the chemical into the water to avoid dangerous chemical reactions.

3. When you are adding more than one chemical to your tub or spa water, do it one chemical at a time. There should be at least a ten-minute interval between the addition of any two chemicals; when adding chlorine and an acid, allow a minimum of one hour between applications.

4. Be very careful not to spill acid on your clothes or skin. Acids can easily burn holes in both.

5. Always dilute any acid in a separate container, then add the diluted solution to your tub water gradually. Be careful not to splash the solution on yourself. Even when it is diluted, acid can damage your clothing or your skin.

6. Chemicals can corrode the metal parts of your support system. Whenever you are adding any chemical to your tub, remember to turn off the primary pump and leave it off until the chemical has mixed thoroughly with the tub water. If you have a blower, you can turn it on to speed up the mixing process.

7. Store all chemicals under lock and key to prevent children from getting at them.

8. Chemicals should be stored in a cool, dry

place. But do not store them in any enclosed space that contains any of the support equipment. The fumes from some chemicals may corrode the metal parts of your equipment.

9. Reread the labels on your chemicals every time you use them, and follow the manufacturer's instructions exactly.

10. Wash thoroughly with soap and water after handling any chemical.

MAINTAINING WOODEN TUBS

The second area of maintenance concerns the tub itself. It should be remembered that wood is a comparatively soft, porous material and as such is subject to unpredictable changes in its shape and texture. Here are suggestions that will extend the life of your tub:

1. Once the tub staves have swelled and are watertight, keep them wet, which means never let the tub stand empty for more than two days. If there are long periods when the tub is not used but the weather is predominantly wet, you can keep it as little as half full, but if the weather is dry, maintain a full amount of water in the tub. The problem you are trying to avoid is that of having the wood dry and shrink, which may twist it out of shape and cause leaks that are nearly impossible to repair.

2. Take good care of the outside of the tub by applying a coat of diluted linseed oil or some other natural preservative to the exterior surfaces. The interior surfaces should never be treated with any sealer so that the water in the tub can penetrate the pores of the wood and keep the staves swollen tightly together.

3. The interior surfaces should be kept clean and smooth. The best way of doing this is to follow a regular water maintenance program that keeps the water in the tub clean.

4. Empty and completely scrub down the inside of the tub every few months, using a garden hose and a brush. Be careful to clean out every nook, such as under the edges of seats and around valve ports.

5. Be aware of the first signs of white streaks in the wood. These will appear as fine, hairlike white cracks in the wood, signifying that too much chlorine or too much acid has begun to break down the cell walls in the wood. The remedy for the streaks is to drain the tub and let the wood dry for a day, then sand the streaks. You can prevent them from appearing again by carefully maintaining your water quality.

6. Prevent rust or corrosion on the metal tub hoops by coating them with a good rust preventative paint or preservative oil two or three times a year.

7. Check for leaks. If any appear after the tub has swelled and is watertight, the cause may be uneven underpinnings. If the tub is not level in all directions, reposition it, then caulk the leaks. If caulking fails to stop the leakage, part or all of the tub may have to be replaced.

MAINTAINING THE SUPPORT SYSTEM

The pump, filter, and heater in your tub support system are all, to one degree or another, mechanical in nature and therefore they require a certain amount of maintenance. It is wise to acquire a maintenance manual for each of the units you own (they usually come with the machinery) and to follow whatever procedures are recommended by the manufacturer.

PUMPS

Generally speaking, pumps and the motors that make them run demand little or no maintenance. Some of them do require lubrication from time to time, but most modern models are sealed for the life of the unit.

You do have to be careful about keeping the prime in the pump. If the pump loses its prime and is allowed to run dry—that is with a lot of air in its chamber—it may overheat and/or damage its water seal. If the pump does lose its prime, the motor should be stopped immediately. Fill the pump with water poured into its leaf strainer basket and replace the basket lid tightly. Then start the motor again.

The leaf strainer should be checked and emptied regularly, particularly in the fall when there is a lot of debris falling from nearby trees. Any time you empty the strainer basket, also check the prime before closing its lid.

HEATERS

About the only problem that arises with heaters is water scale or mineral deposits on the heating elements. Check your heater at least once a year and scrape off any deposits you find on the heating element. If you live in an area with very hard water, you may have to clean the element every six months.

FILTERS

Filters, no matter what they are, require the most care of all, and on the average should be cleaned about once a month. Nearly all filters have pressure gauges that will read between 5 and 10 pounds higher than normal when the filter is dirty or clogged and requires cleaning. Since the filter can become too dirty or too clogged to be of any use at any time of the year, don't rely on regular maintenance to prevent all of your filter problems; check the gauge often and clean the filter whenever necessary.

Diatomaceous Earth (DE) Filters

DE filters are cleaned by backwashing, that is, by reversing the flow of water through them. The immediate result is a loss of filtering material which must then be replaced after you are finished cleaning the filter.

If the DE filter constantly needs cleaning (that is more often than once a month), remove all of the DE and clean the entire unit by hand. Most likely you will discover that the plate which the DE presses against has become clogged.

Sand Filters

These must also be cleaned by backwashing. However, the sand is a permanent part of the filter and will not be lost as it is with a DE filter. If a sand filter seems to require more washing than normal, the sand may have to be washed (or replaced). The most efficient method of doing this is to spend the money to have a pool cleaning contractor do the job for you.

Cartridge Filters

Cartridge filters can always be removed from their units to be cleaned and then replaced—at least for the first year or two. The procedure is simply to pull the cartridge out of its housing, hose and scrub it, and then be sure to replace it correctly so that water can flow through it without being restricted. Be sure to tighten the filter lid properly after you are finished with your cleaning chore.

After one or two years, replace the cartridge, according to the manufacturer's instructions.

PREPARING AND MAINTAINING SPAS

The maintenance of clean water and all of the support system machinery in any spa is identical with that of hot tubs. The start-up procedures and maintenance of the spa surfaces do vary somewhat from those applied to hot tubs. Primarily they are considerably simpler processes.

PREPARING AND MAINTAINING FIBERGLASS SPAS

A fiberglass spa will not leak when you first fill it with water (if it does, return it to the manufacturer). But there will be some residual dust and dirt from the installation, and these must be eliminated before you can have absolutely clean water.

Run your filters from two to four hours a day during the first week after you first fill the spa. Apply spa water clarifiers twice a week and chlorinate more often than is normal until the water is clean and clear.

Once the fiberglass spa is operating at its normal capacity, the major maintenance will be to keep mineral scale, stains, and algae along the water line from driving you nuts. The first line of defense against all of these encroachments is to maintain the proper water condition at all times. In particular, keep the hardness in the water at the lowest possible level by draining the spa frequently and applying the proper water softener.

CLEANING

The spa should be drained every two months or so and completely cleaned. Even before that time, keep a brush nearby and use it to wipe away any stains or algae that may appear at the water line.

After the tub is drained, brush off any scale, dirt, or algae on the surfaces, then wash them with a nonabrasive detergent. If there is a tile band, you can wash it down with a weak solution of muriatic acid (1 part acid to 10 parts water). Use a long-handled soft brush to scrub the tile and wear rubber gloves for your own protection. When the cleaning is completed, hose the inside of the spa thoroughly and then refill it.

Every six months or so you may want to spruce up the finish on the fiberglass by giving it a coating of fiberglass wax available at spa dealers.

CONCRETE SPAS

Concrete spas usually mean Gunite, and Gunite needs some special care during its first few months of use, while the plaster has a chance to cure. Consequently, keep the water in a new Gunite spa clear with extensive filtration and during at least the first four months avoid any heavy chlorination. During the first four-month break-in period, it is best not to add any acid to the water, since even a small amount of acid will etch the plaster before it has had a chance to cure completely.

Gunite spas tend to stain as much as fiberglass, as well as accumulate algae at the water line. After the Gunite has had at least four months to cure properly, the best way of cleaning it is with a 1:10 solution of muriatic acid. But be sure the spa has finished curing before you use any acid at all.

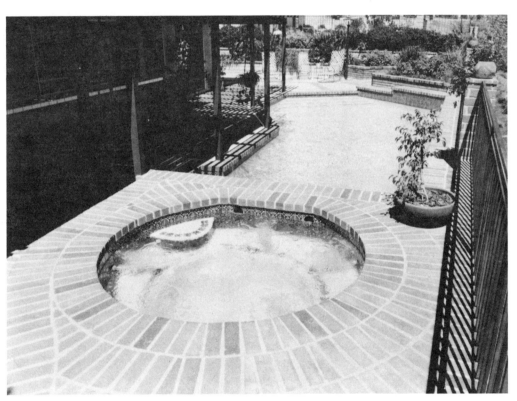

Gunite spas require just as much maintenance as fiberglass and wood.